Bariatric and Metabolic Endoscopy

Editor

RICHARD I. ROTHSTEIN

GASTROINTESTINAL ENDOSCOPY
CLINICS OF NORTH AMERICA

www.giendo.theclinics.com

Consulting Editor
CHARLES J. LIGHTDALE

April 2017 • Volume 27 • Number 2

ELSEVIER

1600 John F. Kennedy Boulevard • Suite 1800 • Philadelphia, Pennsylvania, 19103-2899

http://www.theclinics.com

GASTROINTESTINAL ENDOSCOPY CLINICS OF NORTH AMERICA Volume 27, Number 2
April 2017 ISSN 1052-5157, ISBN-13: 978-0-323-52406-3

Editor: Kerry Holland
Developmental Editor: Donald Mumford

Gastrointestinal Endoscopy Clinics of North America (ISSN 1052-5157) is published quarterly by Elsevier Inc., 360 Park Avenue South, New York, NY 10010-1710. Months of issue are January, April, July, and October. Business and Editorial Offices: 1600 John F. Kennedy Blvd., Suite 1800, Philadelphia, PA, 19103-2899. Periodicals postage paid at New York, NY and additional mailing offices. Subscription prices are $342.00 per year for US individuals, $560.00 per year for US institutions, $100.00 per year for US students and residents, $377.00 per year for Canadian individuals, $662.00 per year for Canadian institutions, $474.00 per year for international individuals, $662.00 per year for international institutions, and $245.00 per year for Canadian and foreign students/residents. To receive student/resident rate, orders must be accompanied by name of affiliated institution, date of term, and the *signature* of program/residency coordinator on institution letterhead. Orders will be billed at individual rate until proof of status is received. Foreign air speed delivery is included in all *Clinics* subscription prices. All prices are subject to change without notice. **POSTMASTER:** Send address change to *Gastrointestinal Endoscopy Clinics of North America*, Elsevier Health Sciences Division, Subscription Customer Service, 3251 Riverport Lane, Maryland Heights, MO 63043. **Customer Service: 1-800-654-2452 (US). From outside the United States, call 1-314-447-8871. Fax: 1-314-447-8029. E-mail: JournalsCustomerService-usa@elsevier.com (for print support) or JournalsOnlineSupport-usa@elsevier.com (for online support).**

Reprints. For copies of 100 or more, of articles in this publication, please contact the Commercial Reprints Department, Elsevier Inc., 360 Park Avenue South, New York, NY 10010-1710. Tel. 212-633-3874; Fax: 212-633-3820; E-mail: reprints@elsevier.com.

Gastrointestinal Endoscopy Clinics of North America is covered in *Excerpta Medica, MEDLINE/PubMed (Index Medicus), and MEDLINE/MEDLARS.*

Contributors

CONSULTING EDITOR

CHARLES J. LIGHTDALE, MD
Professor of Medicine, Division of Digestive and Liver Diseases, Columbia University Medical Center, New York, New York

EDITOR

RICHARD I. ROTHSTEIN, MD
Joseph M. Huber Professor and Chair of Medicine, Senior Associate Dean for Clinical Affairs, Geisel School of Medicine at Dartmouth, Hanover, New Hampshire; Chief Academic Officer, Senior Vice President for Medical Specialties Service Line, Dartmouth-Hitchcock Medical Center, Lebanon, New Hampshire

AUTHORS

MARK J. ANTONINO, MS
Biologist/Regulatory Lead Reviewer, Gastroenterology Devices Branch of the Division of Reproductive Gastro-Renal and Urological Devices, Center for Devices and Radiological Health, U.S. Food and Drug Administration, Silver Spring, Maryland

LOUIS J. ARONNE, MD, FACP, DABOM, FTOS
Sanford I. Weill Professor of Metabolic Research, Comprehensive Weight Control Center, Division of Endocrinology, Diabetes and Metabolism, Weill Cornell Medical College, New York, New York

MARTHA W. BETZ, PhD
Biomedical Engineer/Regulatory Senior Lead Reviewer, Gastroenterology Devices Branch of the Division of Reproductive Gastro-Renal and Urological Devices, Center for Devices and Radiological Health, U.S. Food and Drug Administration, Silver Spring, Maryland

JOEL V. BRILL, MD, FACP, AGAF, FASGE, FACG
Chief Medical Officer, Predictive Health LLC, Paradise Valley; Assistant Clinical Professor of Medicine, University of Arizona College of Medicine, Tucson, Arizona

ALLEN F. BROWNE, MD, FACS, FAAP, Diplomate ABOM
Consulting Pediatric Surgeon, Maine Medical Center, Portland, Maine

ALAN D. CHERRINGTON, PhD
Professor, Molecular Physiology and Biophysics, Jacquelyn A. Turner and Dr. Dorothy J. Turner Chair in Diabetes Research, Department of Medicine, Vanderbilt University School of Medicine, Nashville, Tennessee

JEFFREY W. COOPER, DVM
Veterinary Medical Officer/Branch Chief, Gastroenterology Devices Branch of the Division of Reproductive Gastro-Renal and Urological Devices, Center for Devices and Radiological Health, U.S. Food and Drug Administration, Silver Spring, Maryland

DIANE CORDRAY, VMD
Veterinary Medical Officer/Regulatory Lead Reviewer, Gastroenterology Devices Branch of the Division of Reproductive Gastro-Renal and Urological Devices, Center for Devices and Radiological Health, U.S. Food and Drug Administration, Silver Spring, Maryland

JACQUES DEVIÈRE, MD, PhD
Professor of Medicine and Chairman, Medical-Surgical Department of Gastroenterology, Hepatopancreatology and Digestive Oncology, Erasme Hospital, Université Libre de Bruxelles, Brussels, Belgium

STEVEN A. EDMUNDOWICZ, MD, FASGE
Medical Director, Digestive Health Center, University of Colorado Hospital, Professor of Medicine, University of Colorado School of Medicine, Aurora, Colorado

MARTIN GOLDING, MD
Gastroenterologist/Medical Officer, Gastroenterology Devices Branch of the Division of Reproductive Gastro-Renal and Urological Devices, Center for Devices and Radiological Health, U.S. Food and Drug Administration, Silver Spring, Maryland

ZUBAIDAH NOR HANIPAH, MD
Bariatric and Metabolic Institute, Cleveland Clinic, Cleveland, Ohio; Department of Surgery, Faculty of Medicine and Health Sciences, University Putra Malaysia, Malaysia

LEON I. IGEL, MD, FACP, DABOM
Assistant Professor of Clinical Medicine, Comprehensive Weight Control Center, Division of Endocrinology, Diabetes and Metabolism, Weill Cornell Medical College, New York, New York

LEE M. KAPLAN, MD, PhD
Director, Obesity, Metabolism and Nutrition Institute, Massachusetts General Hospital, Harvard Medical School, Boston, Massachusetts

NITIN KUMAR, MD
Director, Bariatric Endoscopy Institute, Addison, Illinois

REKHA B. KUMAR, MD, MS
Assistant Professor of Medicine, Comprehensive Weight Control Center, Division of Endocrinology, Diabetes and Metabolism, Weill Cornell Medical College, New York, New York

DAVID MAGGS, MD
Chief Medical Officer, Fractyl Laboratories, Inc, Lexington, Massachusetts

APRIL K. MARRONE, PhD, MBA
Chemist/Regulatory Lead Reviewer, Gastroenterology Devices Branch of the Division of Reproductive Gastro-Renal and Urological Devices, Center for Devices and Radiological Health, U.S. Food and Drug Administration, Silver Spring, Maryland

MARIANNA PAPADEMETRIOU, MD
Clinical Fellow, Division of Gastroenterology, New York University School of Medicine, New York, New York

VIOLETA POPOV, MD, PhD
Director of Bariatric Endoscopy, Division of Gastroenterology, NY VA Harbor Healthcare (Manhattan), Assistant Professor of Medicine, New York University School of Medicine, New York, New York

HARITH RAJAGOPALAN, MD, PhD
Co-Founder and Chief Executive Officer, Fractyl Laboratories, Inc, Lexington, Massachusetts

RICHARD I. ROTHSTEIN, MD
Joseph M. Huber Professor and Chair of Medicine, Senior Associate Dean for Clinical Affairs, Geisel School of Medicine at Dartmouth, Hanover, New Hampshire; Chief Academic Officer, Senior Vice President for Medical Specialties Service Line, Dartmouth-Hitchcock Medical Center, Lebanon, New Hampshire

KARTIK SAMPATH, MD
Instructor of Medicine, Gastroenterology Fellow, Section of Gastroenterology and Hepatology, Department of Medicine, Dartmouth-Hitchcock Medical Center, Lebanon; Geisel School of Medicine at Dartmouth, Hanover, New Hampshire

PHILIP R. SCHAUER, MD
Bariatric and Metabolic Institute, Cleveland Clinic, Cleveland, Ohio

JOSHUA S. SILVERSTEIN, PhD
Biomedical Engineer/Regulatory Lead Reviewer, Gastroenterology Devices Branch of the Division of Reproductive Gastro-Renal and Urological Devices, Center for Devices and Radiological Health, U.S. Food and Drug Administration, Silver Spring, Maryland

ANDREW C. STORM, MD
Bariatric Endoscopy Fellow, Division of Gastroenterology, Hepatology and Endoscopy, Brigham and Women's Hospital, Harvard Medical School, Boston, Massachusetts

SHELBY SULLIVAN, MD
Director of the Gastroenterology Metabolic and Bariatric Program, Department of Internal Medicine, University of Colorado School of Medicine, Aurora, Colorado

CHRISTOPHER C. THOMPSON, MD, MHES
Assistant Professor of Medicine, Director of Therapeutic Endoscopy, Division of Gastroenterology, Hepatology and Endoscopy, Brigham and Women's Hospital, Harvard Medical School, Boston, Massachusetts

DEVIKA UMASHANKER, MD, MBA
Fellow of Obesity Medicine, Comprehensive Weight Control Center, Division of Endocrinology, Diabetes and Metabolism, Weill Cornell Medical College, New York, New York

PRIYA VENKATARAMAN-RAO, MD
Pediatric Gastroenterologist/Medical Officer, Gastroenterology Devices Branch of the Division of Reproductive Gastro-Renal and Urological Devices, Center for Devices and Radiological Health, U.S. Food and Drug Administration, Silver Spring, Maryland

Contents

Obesity is a major health crisis resulting in comorbidities such as hypertension, type 2 diabetes, and obstructive sleep apnea. The need for safe and efficacious drugs to help assist with weight loss and reduce cardiometabolic risk factors is great. With several FDA-approved drugs on the market, there is still a great need to develop long-term obesity treatments or noninvasive oral agents to help assist individuals with obesity when used in conjunction with lifestyle modifications.

Sleeve gastrectomy, gastric bypass, gastric banding, and duodenal switch are the most common bariatric procedures performed worldwide. Ninety-five percent of bariatric operations are performed with minimally invasive laparoscopic technique. Perioperative morbidities and mortalities average around 5% and 0.2%, respectively. Long-term weight loss averages around 15% to 25% or about 80 to 100 lbs (40–50 kg). Comorbidities, including type 2 diabetes, hypertension, dyslipidemia, sleep apnea, arthritis, gastroesophageal reflux disease, and nonalcoholic fatty liver disease, improve or resolve after bariatric surgery.

Bariatric surgical procedures, including gastric bypass, vertical sleeve gastrectomy, and biliopancreatic diversion, are the most effective and durable treatments for obesity. In addition, these operations induce metabolic changes that provide weight-independent improvement in type 2 diabetes, fatty liver disease and other metabolic disorders. Initially thought to work by mechanical restriction of food intake or malabsorption of ingested nutrients, these procedures are now known to work through complex changes in neuroendocrine and immune signals emanating from the gut, including peptide hormones, bile acids, vagal nerve activity, and metabolites generated by the gut microbiota, all collaborating to reregulate appetite, food preference, and energy expenditure. Development of less invasive means of achieving these benefits would allow much greater dissemination of effective, gastrointestinal (GI)-targeted therapies for obesity and metabolic disorders. To reproduce the benefits of bariatric surgery, however, these endoscopic procedures and devices will need to mimic the physiological rather than the mechanical effects of these operations.

Weight regain after bariatric surgery is common and can be managed with surgical interventions or less morbid endoscopic techniques. These endoscopic approaches target structural postoperative changes that are associated with weight regain, most notably dilation of the gastrojejunal anastomosis aperture. Purse string suture placement, as well as argon plasma coagulation application to the anastomosis, may result in significant and durable weight loss. Furthermore, various endoscopic approaches may be used to safely and effectively manage other complications of bariatric surgery that may result in poor weight loss or weight regain after surgery, including fistula formation.

Cost-effective therapies to address the growing epidemic of obesity are a leading priority in modern medicine. Intragastric balloons (IGBs) are one such option, with increased effectiveness compared with pharmacotherapy and diet/exercise and a lower rate of adverse events than bariatric surgery. IGBs are endoscopically placed or swallowed space-occupying devices in the stomach. Three IGB systems were approved in 2015 to 2016 by the Food and Drug Administration for use in the United States, with more devices nearing approval. This article reviews the adverse events and efficacy of IGBs, and practice setup, management of common complications, and dietary advice for patients.

Endoscopic gastric plication techniques are effective for weight loss. These procedures offer the potential for higher efficacy than conservative modalities, such as medications and lifestyle modifications, and lower invasiveness than bariatric surgery. Gastric plication techniques include endoscopic sleeve gastroplasty, primary obesity surgery endolumenal, transoral gastroplasty, and plication with the Articulating Endoscopic Circular (ACE) stapler. Currently, primary obesity surgery endolumenal is under review by the US Food and Drug Administration, and endoscopic sleeve gastroplasty is gaining acceptance. Gastric plication procedures, as with any endoscopic bariatric therapy, should be applied in the setting of a multidisciplinary weight management program with long-term follow-up.

This article focuses on the stomach target devices that are currently in various stages of development. Approved intragastric balloons, devices targeting small bowel and aspiration techniques, are described in other contributions to this issue. Bariatric endoscopic devices targeting the stomach directly alter gastric physiology and promote weight loss by potentially changing functional gastric volume, gastric emptying, gastric wall compliance, neurohormonal signaling, and, thereby, satiety. Many stomach-targeting devices are on the horizon for clinical use, and further study will determine the safety and efficacy for clinical use.

Aspiration therapy is a weight loss therapy in the United States for patients with a body mass index between 35 kg/m^2 and 55 kg/m^2. Aspiration therapy allows patients to remove up to one-third of calories consumed at a meal and causes patients to eat fewer calories than prior to starting treatment. Studies demonstrate 14.2% to 21.5% total body weight loss in participants who complete 1 year of treatment and maintenance of weight loss in patients treated for 2 years. Aspiration therapy is a safe and effective new treatment of obesity.

The small bowel is a prime target for bariatric and metabolic endoscopic therapies. New insights into the mechanisms of action of surgical therapies have led to new endoscopic therapies for obesity, type 2 diabetes mellitus, and the metabolic syndrome. The development of endoluminal sleeves that bypass the proximal duodenum have replicated some of the effects of surgical bypass procedures. The endoscopic dual-path enteral bypass has created new treatment options for these conditions. Duodenal mucosal resurfacing offers significant promise for diabetes management. It is hoped that a durable endoscopic therapy for these conditions will be defined and optimized.

The duodenum has become recognized as a metabolic signaling center that is involved in regulating insulin action and, therefore, insulin resistance states such as type 2 diabetes. Bariatric surgery and other manipulations of the upper intestine, in particular the duodenum, have shown that limiting nutrient exposure or contact in this key region exerts powerful metabolic effects. Early human clinical trial data suggest that endoscopic hydrothermal duodenal mucosal resurfacing is well tolerated in human subjects and has an acceptable safety profile. This article describes the rationale for this endoscopic approach and its early human use, including safety, tolerability, and early efficacy.

Obesity in children and adolescents is a severe health, psychosocial, and economic problem. Treatment of obesity should be based on the physiology, biochemistry, and genetics of the disease. Treatment is designed to prevent the comorbidities of obesity and allow a healthy, high-quality, and productive life. Treatment is based on healthy living and usually involves tools such as pharmacotherapy, medical device therapy, and bariatric surgery. Bariatric surgery is not acceptable to most patients, parents, primary care providers, and payers. The most successful treatment of obesity follows a chronic disease model, provides a continuum of care, and involves many different disciplines.

The recent increase in US Food and Drug Administration-approved weight-loss devices has diversified obesity treatment options. The regulatory pathways for endoscopically placed weight-loss devices and considerations for clinical trials are discussed, including the benefit-risk paradigm intended to aid in weight-loss-device trial development. Also discussed is the benefit-risk analysis of recently approved endoscopic devices. A strategic priority of the FDA Center for Devices and Radiological Health is to increase the use of patient input in decision making. Thus, we consider how endoscopic weight-loss devices with profiles similar to those that have been approved may be viewed in a patient preference study.

Intragastric devices may be of benefit to patients who are unable to achieve weight loss through lifestyle modification and pharmaceuticals. With the help of every member of a multidisciplinary team and ongoing commitment from patients, small, practical steps and goals can lead to long-lasting, healthy weight loss.

GASTROINTESTINAL ENDOSCOPY CLINICS OF NORTH AMERICA

THE CLINICS ARE AVAILABLE ONLINE!
Access your subscription at:
www.theclinics.com

Foreword

Bariatric and Metabolic Endoscopy: New Approaches to Obesity and Diabetes

 CrossMark

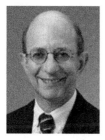

Charles J. Lightdale, MD
Consulting Editor

Each generation of gastrointestinal endoscopists has had unique challenges. For this generation, a major challenge (and opportunity) is to address the huge increase in the incidence of obesity and type 2 diabetes with attendant negative effects on mortality, quality of life, and cost of health care. The root causes of the obesity epidemic are controversial and debatable, but seem to have a relationship to a processed food supply high in sugars and fats, and to a less physically active lifestyle. Certain genetic subgroups may be particularly at risk. Children and adolescents are notably affected, and so dietary and behavioral changes must be applied early. Such interventions coupled with greater public awareness and concern may have blunted the accelerating obesity curve, but there will still be large numbers who require treatment.

There is an obvious need for new approaches. Diet and exercise programs have been effective for only a small minority of the morbidly obese, while pharmaceuticals have been largely ineffective, dangerous, or both. Surgical procedures producing food restriction or malabsorption have worked, but have not had wide acceptance because of risks, side effects, and difficult reversibility. These factors provide the opening for endoscopic innovation, where interventions may be carried out more safely, and offer treatments that can be applied serially in an incremental manner, and often with the possibility of easy reversal. In lessons learned from surgery, a team approach integrating physicians, nurses, dieticians, nutritionists, physical therapists, and psychologists would seem to be helpful.

The editor for this issue of the *Gastrointestinal Endoscopy Clinics of North America* on bariatric and metabolic endoscopy is Dr Richard Rothstein, a valued thought leader in gastrointestinal endoscopy with a futuristic eye, who has been naturally interested in revolutionary endoscopic treatments for obesity and diabetes. He has assembled an outstanding group of expert authors in the field, knowledgeable not only in endoscopy

Gastrointest Endoscopy Clin N Am 27 (2017) xiii–xiv
http://dx.doi.org/10.1016/j.giec.2017.02.001
1052-5157/17/© 2017 Published by Elsevier Inc.

giendo.theclinics.com

but also in the pathophysiology of the derangements associated with obesity and metabolic syndromes. Endoscopic interventions involving the stomach and the small bowel are presented in detail, including options for children and adolescents. Regulatory clearance of novel devices and reimbursement in this evolving area of gastrointestinal endoscopy are additional key topics covered in this issue, which will be of critical importance to researchers and clinicians alike.

This is a state-of-the-art issue and a look to the future for bariatric and metabolic endoscopy. It is also a clarion call for gastrointestinal endoscopists to get off the couch themselves and start thinking about how they may help alleviate the obesity and metabolic syndromes so highly pervasive in our modern society.

Charles J. Lightdale, MD
Department of Medicine
Columbia University Medical Center
161 Fort Washington Avenue
New York, NY 10032, USA

E-mail address:
CJL18@columbia.edu

Preface

Bariatric and Metabolic Endoscopy

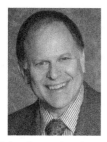

Richard I. Rothstein, MD
Editor

Worldwide, there are approximately 1.3 billion overweight and around 600 million obese individuals. We are experiencing a related rising number of patients with type 2 diabetes mellitus. An alarming number of children and adolescents are overweight or obese, and the plethora of conditions associated with adult obesity is beginning to occur at younger ages. The many causes of obesity are being elucidated, and in the future, precision medicine and targeted therapies will be available for its treatment. In the meantime, we are left with managing weight loss and obesity with available modalities. The standard management of obesity has included lifestyle changes with attention to diet and physical activity, pharmacologic treatment, and surgical intervention. With fewer than 2% of eligible obese individuals choosing to undergo the surgical procedures, and limited efficacy observed from pharmacologic treatments, which have frequent side effects, there is an opportunity for the development and implementation of endoscopic treatments.

A number of endoscopic devices and procedures have been developed to treat obesity and diabetes, and several already have regulatory approval and commercial availability. Others are in clinical or preclinical evaluation, and we await further study in order to determine their role in the growing armamentarium of obesity treatments. Several endoscopic treatments are currently in clinical evaluation for the management of diabetes. In this issue of *Gastrointestinal Endoscopy Clinics of North America*, experts on obesity, diabetes, and the treatments for these conditions provide an update and view to the future, including the status of bariatric and metabolic endoscopy. Initial topics address the current and future medical management of obesity and bariatric surgical interventions. This is followed by a state-of-the-art understanding of body weight and metabolic regulation and what is known about how surgical interventions influence these metabolic processes. Next, a series of articles written by individuals with direct experience highlight the various available and evolving endoscopic devices and techniques and suggest areas of utility and needed iteration. A contribution follows

Gastrointest Endoscopy Clin N Am 27 (2017) xv–xvi
http://dx.doi.org/10.1016/j.giec.2017.01.006
1052-5157/17/© 2017 Published by Elsevier Inc.

giendo.theclinics.com

that reviews the important management of obesity in the pediatric population, including the potential role of endoscopic therapies for this growing cohort. Great ideas and carefully constructed clinical trials will not necessarily result in commercially viable endoscopic solutions that can improve the lives of our patients. The article on regulatory perspectives, written by authors with abundant experience, outlines the various considerations that should be addressed in order to facilitate the regulatory approval of safe and effective devices and therapies. The final contribution on reimbursement perspectives offers superb practical advice from an experienced colleague and outlines pathways of reimbursement strategies for the currently commercially available devices. Comprehensive clinical management by interdisciplinary teams delivering coordinated and longitudinal care is suggested, and billing codes to facilitate payment for standard and endoscopic treatments in evolution are presented.

I want to thank all of the authors in this issue of *Gastrointestinal Endoscopy Clinics of North America* who have generously given their time and expertise so evident in their contributions to this publication. A special thanks to Dr Charlie Lightdale, friend and colleague for so many years, who initiated this issue with the recognition of the importance and timeliness of an update on the current and emerging endoscopic technologies to address obesity and diabetes, and who extended an invitation to edit this collection of work. I appreciate the guidance and assistance of Kerry Holland, Senior Editor, and Donald Mumford, Senior Developmental Editor, at Elsevier, who kept this project moving forward. A thanks to Dartmouth-Hitchcock colleague, Dr Amber Spofford, for the review and editing of the contribution on pediatric treatments. Finally, a thank you to my wife, Lia, who has always provided support and encouragement for my academic career and its myriad responsibilities and activities. I hope you enjoy this issue of *Gastrointestinal Endoscopy Clinics of North America* dedicated to the topic of bariatric and metabolic endoscopy, and I hope that the information presented will be useful as you seek to improve the health of patients with obesity and diabetes in your clinical practice.

Richard I. Rothstein, MD
Dartmouth-Hitchcock Medical Center
Geisel School of Medicine at Dartmouth
1 Medical Center Drive
Lebanon, NH 03756, USA

E-mail address:
richard.rothstein@dartmouth.edu

Current and Future Medical Treatment of Obesity

Devika Umashanker, MD, MBA, Leon I. Igel, MD, Rekha B. Kumar, MD, MS, Louis J. Aronne, MD*

KEYWORDS

- Obesity • Pharmacotherapy • Weight management

KEY POINTS

- Obesity is a public health concern that continues to increase in prevalence in the United States.
- Obesity is a complex disease involving metabolic and neurohormonal processes.
- Several FDA approved drugs work on weight-regulating mechanisms to help with weight loss.

INTRODUCTION

Obesity is a global public health concern that has continued to spread. Epidemiologic data from 2014 reported the prevalence of obesity in the United States to be 35% among men and 40% among women.[1] Compared to 25 years ago when less than 15% of the nation was considered obese.[2] The obesity epidemic has placed an economic burden on the US health care system. The annual medical cost of obesity in the United States was estimated at $147 billion in 2008, with per capita medical expenses 42% higher per person with obesity compared with a person with normal weight.[3] In addition, obesity is associated with job absenteeism costing approximately $4.3 billion annually as well as lower productivity while at work, costing employers $506 per worker with obesity per year.[4,5]

In 2013, obesity was officially recognized as a disease state by the American Medical Association. For adults, the World Health Organization (WHO) defines normal weight as a body mass index (BMI, expressed in kilograms of body weight/height in meters squared) of 18.5 to 24.9 kg/m^2 and overweight as a BMI of 25 to 29.9 kg/m^2. Obesity is further classified into class I for BMI 30 to 34.9 kg/m^2, class II for BMI 35 to 39.9 kg/m^2, and class III for 40 kg/m^2 and above.[6]

Obesity results in many health complications. There are mechanical consequences of increased fat mass and body weight, such as osteoarthritis, obstructive sleep apnea, and urinary incontinence, as well as metabolic consequences due to the hormonal and inflammatory functions of adipose tissue, such as insulin resistance, type II diabetes, cancer, dyslipidemia, hepatosteatosis, and hypertension.[7–12] Tissue inflammation is an

Comprehensive Weight Control Center, Division of Endocrinology, Diabetes, and Metabolism, Weill Cornell Medical College, 1165 York Avenue, New York, NY 10021, USA
* Corresponding author.
E-mail address: ljaronne@mail.med.cornell.edu

Gastrointest Endoscopy Clin N Am 27 (2017) 181–190
http://dx.doi.org/10.1016/j.giec.2016.12.008
1052-5157/17/© 2017 Elsevier Inc. All rights reserved.

Table 1
WHO classification of Body Mass Index

BMI (kg of Body Weight/Height in Meters Squared)	WHO Classification
18.5–24.9	Normal weight
25.0–29.9	Overweight
30.0–34.9	Class 1 obesity
35.0–39.9	Class 2 obesity
40.0 and above	Class 3 obesity

important mechanism linking obesity to insulin resistance in metabolically active organs, such as liver, skeletal muscle, and adipose tissue.[13–15] Adipose tissue is an active endocrine organ that secretes a variety of hormones and proinflammatory cytokines, including leptin, interleukin-6 (IL-6), tumor necrosis factor-alpha (TNF-alpha), resistin, and adiponectin. The adipose tissue–derived hormone leptin exerts its inhibitory effects on food intake primarily by modulating the function of anorectic stimulating neurons in the arcuate nucleus of the hypothalamus.[16] Under conditions of diet-induced obesity, this body of neurons in the hypothalamus becomes resistant to leptin, and as a result, the signaling process for satiety appears to be blunted. Evidence of gliosis in the mediobasal hypothalamus of obese humans, assessed by MRI, suggests neuronal injury in an area crucial for body weight control.[17] Inflammatory markers IL-6 and TNF-alpha as well as resistin secreted by adipocytes promote insulin resistance linked to obesity.[18–21]

Because of counterregulatory neurohormonal mechanisms aimed at maintaining fat mass as a survival measure, weight regain is very common after diet-induced weight loss.[22] Antiobesity pharmacotherapy should be considered as an adjunct to diet and behavioral modification in order to facilitate weight loss or promote long-term weight maintenance. In addition to directly promoting weight loss, antiobesity pharmacotherapy can either directly or indirectly treat comorbid conditions associated with obesity, including prediabetes, type 2 diabetes mellitus (T2D), obstructive sleep apnea, hypertension, and dyslipidemia. Patients and physicians should recognize that expected weight loss from obesity pharmacotherapy is 5% to 10% of total body weight (TBW). For patients with severe obesity (class III), multiple medications or pharmacotherapy in addition to surgical intervention may be considered.

Adjuvant pharmacologic treatments should be considered for patients with a BMI greater than 30 or with a BMI greater than 27 who also have concomitant obesity-related diseases and for whom dietary modifications and physical activity has not been successful.[23] Obesity is a chronic disease requiring continuous management and ongoing interventional efforts, including long-term treatment. Several weight-loss agents have been approved by the US Food and Drug Administration (FDA) for weight management, including phentermine, orlistat, phentermine/topiramate ER, lorcaserin, buproprion/naltrexone, and liraglutide (**Table 1**).

PHENTERMINE

Phentermine was approved by the FDA in 1959 and has been the most commonly prescribed short-term (up to 12 weeks) medication for weight loss. Phentermine is primarily a noradrenergic and possibly dopaminergic sympathomimetic amine.[46] The standard adult dose is up to 37.5 mg daily before breakfast. However, dosages should be individualized to achieve adequate response with the lowest effective dose. A quarter tablet (9.375 mg) or a half tablet (18.75 mg) may be adequate for some patients. A 28-week, randomized, controlled trial compared phentermine 7.5 mg, phentermine 15 mg, topiramate ER 46 mg, topiramate ER 92 mg, with a combination of phentermine and topiramate ER 7.5/46 mg and 15/92 mg. Primary endpoints were percent weight loss and achievement of ≥5% weight loss. Focusing on the phentermine monotherapy arm of the study, individuals taking phentermine 7.5 mg daily and 15 mg daily lost 5.3 kg and 6.0 kg, respectively, compared with 1.5 kg for placebo.[24] The percentage of subjects achieving ≥5% weight loss was 15.5% for placebo, 43.3% for phentermine 7.5 mg, and 46.6% for phentermine 15 mg.[24] Potential side effects of phentermine include dizziness, dry mouth, difficulty sleeping, and irritability.

ORLISTAT (XENICAL)

Orlistat was approved in 1999 by the FDA for weight management in conjunction with reduced calorie diet. Orlistat alters fat digestion by inhibiting gastric and pancreatic lipases, causing approximately 30% fecal fat excretion. Orlistat is prescribed 3 times a day at a dosage of 120 mg to be taken with meals. A lower-dose formulation containing 60 mg per capsule is available over the counter and sold under the brand name Alli.

Several randomized trials have demonstrated the efficacy of orlistat in promoting weight loss. The 4-year XENDOS (Xenical in the Prevention of Diabetes in Obese Subjects) study demonstrated a 5.8-kg weight loss in the orlistat group (120 mg taken 3 times per day) compared with a 3.0-kg weight loss in the placebo group. After 4 years, 52.8% of the patients in the orlistat group had lost ≥5% of TBW and 26.2% of subjects had lost ≥10% TBW.[47] The Xendos study also demonstrated reduced progression from impaired glucose tolerance to overt T2D. The progression of prediabetes to diabetes was seen in 6.2% of the orlistat group compared with 9.0% of subjects in the placebo group; a 42% reduction.[47]

Side effects of orlistat include bloating, flatulence, flatus with discharge, and fecal incontinence. Because orlistat may reduce the absorption of fat-soluble vitamins (A, D, E, K), a multivitamin supplement is advised when treating with this agent.

LORCASERIN (BELVIQ)

Lorcaserin was approved by the FDA in 2012 for long-term weight management. Lorcaserin is a selective serotonin 2c receptor agonist. Lorcaserin decreases food consumption and promotes satiety by selectively activating the 5HT-2c receptor on anorexigenic POMC neurons located in the hypothalamus.[23] At the recommended daily dose of 10 mg twice a day, lorcaserin selectively interacts with 5-HT2c receptors as opposed to 5-HT2a and 5HT2b, which have been implicated in the risk of both depression and cardiac valve insufficiency, respectively.[25]

Three randomized, double-blinded, placebo-controlled studies were conducted to evaluate the efficacy of lorcaserin on weight loss: BLOOM (Behavioral Modification and Lorcaserin for Overweight and Obesity Management), BLOSSOM (Behavioral Modification and Lorcaserin Second Study for Obesity Management), and BLOOM-DM performed specifically in adults with T2D.

The BLOOM trial included 3182 patients with obesity or overweight who were randomized to receive lorcaserin 10 mg twice a day or placebo for 52 weeks, along with diet and exercise counseling. Primary outcomes were weight loss at 52 weeks and weight maintenance at 104 weeks. At 52 weeks, the lorcaserin group lost 5.8 kg compared with 2.2 kg in the placebo group.[25] The percentage of patients taking lorcaserin who achieved TBW loss of ≥5% TBW at year 1 was 47% compared with 20.5% of the placebo group.[25] At 52 weeks, patients in the lorcaserin group were randomly reassigned to receive treatment or placebo for another 52 weeks. Among patients in the lorcaserin group, those who continued to receive lorcaserin had better maintenance of weight loss compared with those who were reassigned to receive placebo.

The most common adverse effects seen in patients on lorcaserin are headaches, dizziness, and nausea.[26] The most common side effect noted in patients with T2D on lorcaserin was symptomatic hypoglycemia, requiring a reduction in diabetic medication dosage.[27,28]

PHENTERMINE/TOPIRAMATE ER (QSYMIA)

A low-dose, fixed-release capsule combining extended release phentermine and topiramate was approved by the FDA in 2012 as adjuvant therapy for individuals with obesity or overweight with at least one comorbid condition. Phentermine increases norepinephrine in the hypothalamus, enhancing POMC neuron pathway signaling to increase alpha-MSH, which binds to melanocortin 4 receptor and suppresses appetite.[25] The exact mechanism of action for weight loss with topiramate is not known, although animal studies suggest that topiramate-induced weight loss results from increased energy expenditure, decreased energetic efficiency, and decreased caloric intake as an appetite suppressant.[29,42,43] Phentermine/Topiramate ER comes in 4 dosages: 3.75/23 mg (starting dose), 7.5/46 mg (treatment dose) 11.25/69 mg, or 15/92 mg (maximum dose). Phentermine/Topiramate ER is initiated through a stepwise approach, starting at 3.75/23 mg once daily for 2 weeks before increasing to the recommended dose of 7.5/46 mg once daily.[30] Further titration to a maximum dose of 15/92 mg once daily may be considered for individuals who do not achieve 3% weight loss after 12 weeks.[31] If 5% weight loss is not achieved after 12 weeks at 15/92 mg per day, then phentermine/topiramate ER dose should be gradually reduced for discontinuation.[30]

The CONQUER trial, a 1-year double-blinded, placebo-controlled study of 2487 adults whom are overweight or obese with 2 or more comorbidities were randomized to receive phentermine/topiramate ER 7.5/46 mg, phentermine/topiramate ER15/92 mg or placebo. At 1 year, both groups assigned to active treatment had significantly greater weight loss than the placebo group. In the phentermine/topiramate ER 7.5/46 mg and phentermine/topiramate 15/92 mg arms of the study, 62% and 70% of patients, respectively, lost ≥5% TBW compared with 21% with placebo.[25] SEQUEL was a 108-week extension study in which participants who completed the CONQUER study continued their previously assigned treatment. Patients in both active treatment arms experienced greater weight loss compared with those in the placebo arm. Phentermine/Topiramate ER 7.5/46 mg had a 9.6-kg weight loss and phentermine/topiramate 15/92 mg had a 10.9-kg weight loss from baseline compared with 2.1-kg weight loss with placebo.[25] In addition, 75% of the phentermine/topiramate ER 7.5/46-mg group and 79.3% of the phentermine/topiramate 15/92-mg group achieved ≥5% weight loss compared with 30% of the placebo-treated patients.[25] In all groups treated with phentermine/topiramate ER, greater reductions in systolic blood pressure, hemoglobin A1c, prediabetes, low-density lipoprotein cholesterol, triglycerides, and waist circumference were seen compared with placebo.

The most common side effects noted with phentermine/topiramate ER were paresthesias, dizziness, dysgeusia, and dry mouth. The FDA required a Risk Evaluation and Mitigation Strategy for phentermine/topiramate ER to inform women of reproductive age about the increased risk of congenital malformation, specifically orofacial clefts, in infants exposed to the topiramate component of the drug during the first trimester of pregnancy.

LIRAGLUTIDE 3.0 (SAXENDA)

Liraglutide 3.0, a glucagon-like peptide-1 (GLP-1) agonist, is FDA approved for chronic weight management in individuals with obesity. GLP-1 agonists cause glucose-dependent insulin secretion from pancreatic beta cells to lower glucose levels (primary mechanism of use in diabetes), suppression of glucagon secretion, and slowing of gastric emptying. Originally developed as a treatment option for patients with T2D in 2010, liraglutide, under the brand name Victoza, was approved at doses up to 1.8 mg once daily. Liraglutide 3.0 was FDA approved in 2014 to be used at doses up to 3.0 mg once daily for the treatment of individuals with BMI ≥ 30 or BMI ≥ 27 with comorbidities. SCALE Diabetes, a 56-week, randomized, double-blinded clinical trial, was performed in 846 patients with T2D and either overweight or obesity to assess the efficacy of liraglutide 3 mg for weight loss in conjunction with lifestyle modification. At 56 weeks, adults treated with liraglutide 3 mg achieved significantly greater weight loss (5.9%) compared with placebo (2.0%).[25] SCALE Obesity and Prediabetes, a study involving patients with obesity or overweight without diabetes assessed the efficacy of liraglutide 3 mg and found that, after 56 weeks patients receiving liraglutide 3 mg showed significantly greater loss of body weight from baseline (8.0%) compared with those receiving placebo (2.6%).[25] The proportion of patients losing greater than 5% and 10% of body weight with liraglutide 3 mg was 64% and 33%, respectively, compared with those receiving placebo (27% and 10%, respectively).[25]

Notable secondary findings included reduced incidence of type II diabetes, improved systolic blood pressure, reduction in lipids, and reduction in waist circumference.

The most common side effects experienced with liraglutide 3 mg were nausea, vomiting, and diarrhea.[30]

NALTREXONE ER/BUPROPION ER (CONTRAVE)

Naltrexone ER/Bupropion ER (NB) was FDA approved for the treatment of obesity in 2014. Bupropion, used as an antidepressant and to assist with smoking cessation, also has weight-loss effects. Bupropion stimulates hypothalamic POMC neurons, with downstream effects to reduce food intake and increase energy expenditure.[25] Naltrexone blocks opioid receptor–mediated POMC autoinhibition, augmenting POMC firing in a synergistic manner.[25] Given the known individual effects of naltrexone and bupropion on addiction (alcohol and smoking, respectively), a fixed combination NB was hypothesized to induce weight loss through sustained modulation of central nervous system reward pathways.[25]

Four 56-week multicenter, double-blinded, placebo-controlled trials, Contrave Obesity Research I (COR-I), Contrave Obesity Research II (COR-II), Contrave Obesity Research Behavioral Modification (COR-BMOD), and Contrave Obesity Research Diabetes (COR Diabetes), enrolled patients with obesity and overweight with comorbidities. The primary end points of COR-I and COR-II were the percentage of patients losing ≥5% TBW with the combination formulation compared with placebo. At week 56 in COR-I, the mean change in body weight with NB 16/360 mg and NB 32/360 mg was 5% and 6.1%, respectively, compared with 1.3% with placebo.[25] After 56 weeks in the COR-BMOD study, patients on Contrave + BMOD had a significant reduction in body weight (−11.5%) compared with BMOD alone (−7.3%).[25] COR-Diabetes was conducted to study the efficacy and safety profile of NB in patients with T2D and either overweight or obese. Of patients taking NB, 44.5% achieved greater than 5% weight loss compared with 18.9% of placebo group.[25]

Evaluation of secondary endpoints demonstrated increased high-density lipoprotein (HDL) cholesterol, reduction of triglycerides, reduction in both systolic and diastolic blood pressure, and reduction in waist circumference.[25] In addition, the NB 32/360 mg group had a reduction of fasting glucose and insulin levels.[25] In the COR-II study, improvements were noted in lipid profile, systolic blood pressure, and waist circumference but not in diastolic blood pressure or fasting glucose.[25] In the

COR-BMOD trial, there were significant changes with NB + BMOD compared with placebo + BMOD in HDL cholesterol, triglycerides, fasting insulin, and waist circumference. Changes in blood pressure were not assessed.[25] In COR-Diabetes, NB treatment was associated with improvements in glycemic control, HDL cholesterol, and triglycerides compared with placebo (**Table 2**).[25]

Antidiabetic Medications That Promote Weight Loss

Over the past 32 years, from 1980 through 2012, the number of adults diagnosed with diabetes in the United States has nearly quadrupled, from 5.5 million to 21.3 million.[44] Among adults, about 1.7 million new cases of diabetes are diagnosed each year.[44] There are several diabetes drugs available that promote modest weight loss, including Metformin, SGLT2 inhibitors, GLP-1 agonists, and pramlintide.

Metformin (a biguanide derivative) is the first-line pharmacologic therapy for patients with T2D and can be useful in preventing or delaying diabetes in patients with prediabetes, defined as hemoglobin A1C from 5.7% to 6.4%.[32] Metformin is a valuable therapy for most patients with T2D due to its high rate of efficacy, low risk of hypoglycemia, and low cost.

Metformin reduces serum glucose levels by several different mechanisms, notably through nonpancreatic mechanisms without increasing insulin secretion. Metformin suppresses the endogenous glucose production by the liver, which is mainly due to a reduction in the rate of gluconeogenesis and a small effect on glycogenolysis, decreases the peripheral uptake of glucose, and increases the peripheral glucose disposal that arises largely through increased nonoxidative glucose disposal into skeletal muscle.[31,33,34]

The Diabetes Prevention Program, a large-scale trial involving 3234 patients with impaired glucose tolerance, primarily evaluated the incidence of diabetes at the end of the treatment period among patients treated with either Metformin, standard lifestyle intervention (placebo group), or intensive lifestyle modification. After an average of 2.8 years of follow-up, the metformin-treated group lost 2.5% of their body weight compared with placebo.[35,36]

The most common side effects of metformin are gastrointestinal, including a metallic taste in the mouth, mild anorexia, nausea, abdominal discomfort, diarrhea, or rarely, lactic acidosis.[35]

Sodium glucose transporter 2 inhibitors

A new class of antidiabetic drugs that have an impact on weight loss involves the sodium glucose cotransporter inhibitors (SGLT2I), and canagliflozin, dapagliflozin, and empagliflozin. The mechanism of action of the selective inhibitors of SGLT2 is to reduce glucose reabsorption, causing excess glucose to be eliminated in the urine,

Table 2
Common Adverse effects of US Food and Drug Administration–approved weight loss medications

Agent	Common Adverse Effects
Phentermine	Dizziness, dry mouth, difficulty sleeping, irritability
Orlistat	Flatus with discharge, oily spotting, bloating
Lorcaserin	Non–diabetes mellitus: Headache, fatigue, nausea, dry mouth Diabetes mellitus: hypoglycemia, back pain, fatigue
Phentermine/Topiramate ER	Paresthesia, dysgeusia, Insomnia, dizziness
Naltrexone ER/Buproprion ER	Nausea, constipation, headache, vomiting
Liraglutide 3.0 mg	Diarrhea, constipation, dyspepsia

which results in a decrease in plasma glucose levels. The glucosuria produced by the SGLTT2 inhibitors is associated with weight loss, and the diuretic effect causes a decrease in blood pressure.

The initial dose for canagliflozin is 100 mg daily taken before breakfast, which can be increased to 300 mg daily. Initial dosage of dapagliflozin is 5 mg, which can be increased to 10 mg daily. Empagliflozin initial dosage is10 mg once daily, which can also be increased to 25 mg once daily.

A direct and network meta-analysis was conducted to evaluate the efficacy of SGLT2 I as weight-loss medications for patients with T2D who have been on an SGLT2 I for at least 12 weeks. The review demonstrated SGLT2-I to help with weight loss. Patients on canagliflozin 300 mg, empagliflozin 25 mg, and dapagliflozin 10 mg had a mean weight loss of 2.66 kg, 1.81 kg, and 1.80 kg, respectively, when compared with placebo.[44] In 2015, the Empagliflozin Cardiovascular Outcome Event Trial in Type 2 Diabetes Mellitus study demonstrated individuals with Type 2 Diabetes on Empagliflozin with high cardiovascular risk had reduced cardiac primary endpoints (nonfatal stroke, CV death, and nonfatal myocardial infarction) and reduction in heart failure hospitalizations.

Most common side effects of SGLT2 inhibitors include yeast infection and urinary tract infections.

Glucagon-like Polypeptide-1 agonists
Another class of antidiabetic drugs that promote weight loss is the GLP-1 agonists, which include exenatide (Byetta), exenatide XR (Bydureon), albiglutide (Tanzeum) and dulaglutide (Trulicity) and liraglutide (Victoza). GLP-1s are gastrointestinal peptides secreted from the ileum and jejunum that stimulate glucose-dependent insulin secretion and inhibit glucagon release and gastric emptying. Unlike exenatide XR, which is administered subcutaneously 2 mg once weekly, exenatide is administered subcutaneously 10 µg twice daily. Liraglutide (Victoza), another GLP-1 analogue, is used for the treatment of T2D at a maximum dose of 1.8 mg once daily.

A randomized trial over 30 weeks involving 295 patients was conducted to evaluate the safety and efficacy of once-weekly exenatide Long Acting Release (LAR) versus twice daily exenatide. During this trial, a progressive reduction in body weight was observed throughout the study with both treatment groups experiencing similar reductions in weight from baseline (−3.7 kg with exenatide LAR vs −3.6 kg with twice daily exenatide).[45] In 2016, the Liraglutide Effect and Action in Diabetes: Evaluation of Cardiovascular Outcome Result (LEADER) study revealed liraglutide (Victoza) had significant effects in reducing the rates of major adverse cardiovascular events in type 2 diabetes patients at elevated cardiovascular risk.

The most frequent side effects include nausea and vomiting.[45]

Pramlintide (Symlin)
Pramlintide, an analogue of the pancreatic hormone amylin, is approved to assist glycemic control in type 1 diabetes and T2D patients taking insulin. Pramlintide is secreted with insulin by pancreatic beta cells in response to food intake. Pramlintide can be administered at doses of 30–120 µg 3 times per day with meals.

In one study, 204 people with obesity were randomly assigned to take 120 µg of pramlintide or a placebo 3 times a day before meals for 4 months. Both groups received lifestyle interventions aimed at weight loss. A greater percentage of the pramlintide group (31%) lost 5% or more of their body weight compared with 2% of the placebo group, and a substantially higher percentage of people in the pramlintide group reported better appetite control and improved well-being.[37–39]

The most common side effects of pramlintide are hypoglycemia, nausea, followed by anorexia and vomiting.[38]

Future Option for Obesity Pharmacotherapy

Gelesis 100

Gelesis 100 is a novel oral capsule device designed to achieve weight loss in adults who are overweight or have obesity, including those with prediabetes and T2D.[38] Each capsule contains thousands of proprietary, biocompatible hydrogel particles synthesized with starting materials that are Generally Recognized as Safe by the FDA.[40] Gelesis 100 capsules are taken before a meal with water, after which the small particles within the capsules hydrate and expand in the stomach and small intestine, triggering several important satiety and glycemic control mechanisms. Gelesis 100 has several built-in safety features: (a) the volume it creates is limited by the amount of water consumed; (b) the hydrated particles, which are 2 mm in size, do not cluster or stick together and have similar elasticity (rigidity) as ingested food; and (c) the particles partially degrade in the colon, releasing absorbed water.[41]

The GLOW (Gelesis Loss of Weight) trial received positive confirmation from the FDA in July 2015, allowing gelesis to expand the study to multiple US sites.[38] The primary endpoints are to evaluate change in TBW from baseline to end of treatment, and percentage of individuals with at least 5% weight loss. The secondary endpoints include changes in key glycemic control parameters.[41]

SUMMARY

Obesity is a major health crisis resulting in comorbidities such as hypertension, T2D, and obstructive sleep apnea. The need for safe and efficacious drugs to help assist with weight loss and reduce cardiometabolic risk factors is great. With several FDA-approved drugs now on the market, there is still a great need to develop additional obesity pharmacotherapies, or noninvasive oral agents, to assist individuals with overweight/obesity when used in conjunction with lifestyle modification.

REFERENCES

1. Flegal KM, Kruszon-Moran D, Carroll MD, et al. Trends in obesity among adults in the United States, 2005 to 2014. JAMA 2016;315(21):2284–91.
2. State of obesity, Better policies for healthier America. Available at: http://stateofobesity.org/. Accessed September 17, 2015.
3. Finkelstein EA, Trogdon JG, Cohen JW, et al. Annual medical spending attributable to obesity: payer-and service-specific estimates. Health Aff 2009;28(5):w822–31.
4. Cawley J, Rizzo JA, Haas K. Occupation-specific absenteeism costs associated with obesity and morbid obesity. J Occup Environ Med 2007;49(12):1317–24.
5. Gates D, Succop P, Brehm B, et al. Obesity and presenteeism: the impact of body mass index on workplace productivity. J Occup Environ Med 2008;50(1):39–45.
6. WHO Obesity and Overweight Fact sheets 2016. Available at: http://www.who.int/mediacentre/factsheets/fs311/en/. Accessed September 17, 2015.
7. Garvey WT, Garber AJ, Mechanick JI, et al. American Association of Clinical Endocrinologists and American College of Endocrinology consensus conference on obesity: building and evidence base for comprehensive action. Endocr Pract 2014;20:956–76.
8. Garber AJ, Abrahamson MJ, Barzilay JI, et al. American Association of Clinical Endocrinologists comprehensive diabetes management algorithm 2013 consensus statement. Endocr Pract 2013;19:1–48.

9. Jensen MD, Ryan DH, Apovian CM, et al. 2013 AHA/ACC/TOS guideline for the management of overweight and obesity in adults: a report of the American College of Cardiology/American Heart Association Task Force on Practice Guidelines and The Obesity Society. J Am Coll Cardiol 2014;63(25 Pt B):2985-3023.

10. Seger JC, Horn DB, Westman EC, et al. Obesity Algorithm, present by the American Society of Bariatric Physicians. Available at: http://www.asbp.org/obeistyalgorithm.html. Accessed March 10, 2015.

11. Pi-Sunyer X. The medical risks of obesity. Postgrad Med 2009;121:21-33.

12. Roux L, Kuntz KM, Donaldson C, et al. Economic evaluation of weight loss interventions in overweight and obese women. Obesity (Silver Spring) 2006;14:1093-106.

13. Lumeng CN, Saltiel AR. Inflammatory links between obesity and metabolic disease. J Clin Invest 2011;121(6):2111-7.

14. Schenk S, Saberi M, Olefsky JM. Insulin sensitivity; modulation by nutrients and inflammation. J Clin Invest 2008;118(9):2992-3002.

15. Shoelson SE, Lee J, Goldfine AB. Inflammation and insulin resistance. J Clin Invest 2006;116(7):1793-801.

16. Lee E, Ahima RS. Alteration of hypothalamic cellular dynamics in obesity. J Clin Invest 2012;122(1):22-5.

17. Thaler JP, Yi CX, Schur EA, et al. Obesity is associated with hypothalamic injury in rodents and humans. J Clin Invest 2012;122(1):153-62.

18. Scherer PE, Williams S, Fogliano M, et al. A novel serum protein similar to c1q produced exclusively in adipocytes. J Biol Chem 1995;270:26746-9.

19. Snehalatha C, Mukesh B, Simon M, et al. Plasma adiponectin is an independent predictor of type 2 diabetes in Asian Indians. Diabetes Care 2003;26:3226-9.

20. Halperin F, Beckman JA, Patti ME, et al. The role of total and high molecular-weight complex of adiponectin in vascular function in offspring whose parents both had type 2 diabetes. Diabetologia 2005;48:2147-54.

21. Kadowaki T, Yamauchi T, Kubota N, et al. Adiponectin and adiponectin receptors in insulin resistance, diabetes, and the metabolic syndrome. J Clin Invest 2006;116:1784-92.

22. Kumar RB, Aronne LJ. Efficacy comparison of medications approved for chronic weight management. Obesity (Silver Spring) 2015;23(Suppl 1):S4-7.

23. Kushner R, Lawrence V, Kumar S. Practical manual of clinical obesity. USA: John Wiley & Sons, LTD; 2013.

24. Aronne LJ, Wadden TA, Peterson C, et al. Evaluation of phentermine and topiramate versus phentermine/topiramate extended release in obese adults. Obesity 2013;21:2163-71.

25. Apovian C, Aronne L, Powell A. Clinical management of obesity. 1st edition. New York: Professional Communications Inc; 2015.

26. Courcoulas AP, Christian NJ, Belle SH, et al, Longitudinal Assessment of Bariatric Surgery (LABS) Consortium. Weight change and health outcomes at 3 years after bariatric surgery among individuals with severe obesity. JAMA 2013;310:2416-25.

27. Smith SR, Weissman NJ, Anderson CM, et al. Multicenter, placebo-controlled trial of lorcaserin for weight management. N Engl J Med 2010;363:245.

28. O'Neil PM, Smith SR, Weissman NJ, et al. Randomized placebo-controlled clinical trial of lorcaserin for weight loss in type 2 DM: the BLOOM-DM study. Obesity (Silver Spring) 2012;20:1426.

29. Richard D, Ferland J, Lalonde J, et al. Influence of topiramate in the regulation of energy balance. Nutrition 2000;16(10):961-6.

30. US Food and Drug Admistration. Drugs@FDA: FRA approved drug products (product specific prescribing information). Available at: http://www.accessdata.fda.gov/Scripts/cder/DrugsatFDA/. Accessed March 10, 2015.

31. Effect of intensive blood glucose control with Metformin on complications in overweight patients with Type 2 diabetes (UKPDS 34). UK Prospective Diabetes Study (UKPDS) Group. Lancet 1998;352(9131):854–65.

32. American Diabetes Association. Standards of medical care in diabetes, 2014. Diabetes Care 2014;37(Suppl 1):S14–80.

33. Seo-Mayer PW, Thulin G, Zhang L, et al. Preactivation of AMPK by metformin may ameliorate the epithelial cell damage caused by renal ischemia. Am J Physiol Renal Physiol 2011;301:F1346–57.

34. Rosen P, Wiernsperger NF. Metformin delays the manifestation of diabetes and vascular disfunction in Goto-Kakizaki rats by reduction of mitochondrial oxidative stress. Diabetes Metab Res Rev 2006;22:323–30.

35. Glandt M, Raz I. Present and future: pharmacologic treatment of obesity. J Obes 2011;2011:636181.

36. Knolwer WC, Barrett-Connor E, Fowler SE, et al. Reduction in the incidence of type 2 diabetes with lifestyle intervention or metformin. N Engl J Med 2002;346(6):393–403.

37. Aronne L, Fujioka K, Aroda V, et al. Progressive reduction in body weight after treatment with the amylin analog pramlintide in obese subjects: a phase 2, randomized, placebo controlled, dose escalation study. J Clin Endocrinol Metab 2007;92(8):2977–83.

38. Smith SR, Aronne LJ, Burns CM, et al. Sustained weight loss following 12 month pramlintide treatment as an adjunct to lifestyle intervention in obesity. Diabetes Care 2008;31(9):1816–23.

39. Diabetes 2014 Report Card, Center for Disease Control and Prevention. Available at: https://www.cdc.gov/diabetes/library/reports/reportcard.html. Accessed October 1, 2016.

40. "Gelesis Enrolls first US patient in GLOW Gelesis 100 trial". 2016. Available at: BariatricNews.net. Accessed September 29, 2016.

41. "Gelesis Announces Initiation of a Six-Month Weight Loss Study with Gelesis100". 2015. Available at: PRNnews.com. Accessed September 9, 2016.

42. Richard D, Picard F, Lemieux C, et al. The effects of topiramate and sex hormones on energy balance of male and female rats. Int J Obes Relat Metab Disord 2002;26(3):344–53.

43. Picard F, Deshaies Y, Lalonde J, et al. Topiramate reduces energy and fat gains in lean (Fa/FA) and obese (fa/fa) Zucker rats. Obes Res 2000;8(9):656–63.

44. Pinto LC, Rados DV, Remonti LR, et al. Efficacy of SGLT2 inhibitors in glycemic control, weight loss and blood pressure reduction: a systematic review and meta-analysis. Diabetol Metab Syndr 2015;7(Suppl 1).

45. Garber AJ. Long acting glucagon-like peptide 1 receptor agonists: review of their efficacy and tolerability. Diabetes Care 2011;34:S279–84.

46. Apovian CM, Aronne LJ, Bessesen DH, et al. Pharmacological management of obesity: an endocrine society clinical practice guideline. J Clin Endocrinol Metab 2015;100(2):342–62.

47. Togerson JS, Haupman J, Boldrin MN, et al. In the prevention of diabetes in obese subject (XENDOS) study; a randomized study of orlistat as an adjunct to lifestyle changes for the prevention of type 2 diabetes in obese patient. Diabetes Care 2004;27(1):155–61.

Surgical Treatment of Obesity and Diabetes

 CrossMark

Zubaidah Nor Hanipah, MD[a,b], Philip R. Schauer, MD[a,*]

KEYWORDS

- Bariatric surgery • Metabolic surgery • Obesity • Weight loss • Diabetes

KEY POINTS

- Sleeve gastrectomy, gastric bypass, gastric banding, and duodenal switch are the most common bariatric procedures performed worldwide.
- Ninety-five percent of bariatric operations are performed with minimally invasive laparoscopic technique.
- Perioperative morbidities and mortalities average around 5% and 0.2%, respectively.
- Long-term weight loss averages around 15% to 25% or about 80 to 100 lbs (40–50 kg).
- Comorbidities, including type 2 diabetes, hypertension, dyslipidemia, sleep apnea, arthritis, gastroesophageal reflux disease, and nonalcoholic fatty liver disease, improve or resolve after bariatric surgery.

INTRODUCTION

Bariatric surgery has evolved since the 1950s and has proven to be the most effective long-term treatment for the chronic disease known as obesity. Furthermore, it also has been shown to resolve or significantly improve many of the metabolic disorders related to obesity, especially type 2 diabetes (T2D). These gastrointestinal procedures have resulted in resolution of obesity-related comorbidities through weight loss, neuroendocrine, or hormonal mechanisms. Thus, the term bariatric surgery is now frequently replaced with metabolic surgery. A complete understanding of all the mechanisms of metabolic surgery is yet to be determined. It is known, however, that the alteration of the gastrointestinal tract by reducing stomach capacity and nutrient absorption in the small intestine alters the satiety, calorie absorption, and neuroendocrine pathways, leading to sustained weight loss and resolution of T2D.[1]

Disclosure Statement: The authors have nothing to disclose.
[a] Bariatric and Metabolic Institute, Digestive Disease and Surgical Institute, Cleveland Clinic, 9500 Euclid Avenue, Cleveland, OH 44022, USA; [b] Department of Surgery, Faculty of Medicine and Health Sciences, University Putra Malaysia, UPM-Serdang, 43400 Serdang, Selangor, Malaysia
* Corresponding author. Cleveland Clinic, 9500 Euclid Avenue, M61, Cleveland, OH 44022.
E-mail address: schauep@ccf.org

The laparoscopic technique of bariatric/metabolic surgery was started in the early 1990s, and currently, almost 95% of these metabolic procedures are performed laparoscopically worldwide. The laparoscopic approach significantly reduces perioperative morbidity, mortality, recovery time, and cost.[2] In 2015, a total of 196,000 bariatric/metabolic procedures were performed in the United States, and sleeve gastrectomy (SG) was the commonest metabolic procedure (53.8%). Other metabolic procedures were Roux-en-Y gastric bypass (RYGB), 23.1%; laparoscopic adjustable gastric band (LAGB), 5.7%; biliopancreatic diversion with or without duodenal switch (BPD ± DS), 0.6%; and revisional and other procedures, 16.8%.[3]

Bariatric surgery was initially introduced as weight-loss surgery for the treatment of severe obesity. Obesity is most commonly measured based on body mass index (BMI), which has been used as the primary indication for bariatric surgery. The 1991 National Institutes of Health (NIH),[4] 2013 American College of Cardiology/American Heart Association Task Force, and The Obesity Society (TOS)[5] have similar guidelines for bariatric surgery referral: BMI greater than or equal to 40 kg/m^2 or BMI greater than or equal to 35 kg/m^2 with obesity-related comorbidities. It is becoming increasingly evident that BMI itself is not necessarily a strong marker for obesity-related illness or future cardiovascular risk. It appears that fat distribution and quantity of visceral fat rather than BMI alone convey the major risk factors for obesity.[6] Metabolic surgery in patients with T2D should be tailored based on the class of obesity and inadequate glycemic control despite optimal medical treatment. Based on strong evidence from randomized trials, metabolic surgery was recently recommended in the treatment algorithm for T2D in the 2nd Diabetes Surgery Summit (DSS-II).[7]

PATIENT SELECTION FOR METABOLIC SURGERY

Indications for bariatric surgery are based on the historic 1991 NIH Consensus Guidelines.[4] These guidelines focused primarily on surgery as treatment of severe obesity, but not necessarily for those with T2D and obesity-related metabolic diseases. In general, patients with chronic obesity and BMI greater than or equal to 40 or BMI greater than or equal to 35 with comorbidity are candidates for surgery if they are psychologically stable and have no active substance abuse. Recently, the DSS-II in collaboration with 6 International Diabetes Organizations published a joint statement on the treatment algorithm for T2D using metabolic surgery.[7] This joint statement was endorsed by 45 leading professional societies worldwide (including both medical and surgical organizations). The indications and contraindications for metabolic surgery are shown in **Table 1**.

Metabolic surgery should be performed in high-volume centers with a multidisciplinary team (including the surgeon, endocrinologist/diabetologist, and dietician with expertise in diabetes care). Other relevant specialists should be considered depending on the patients' circumstances.

Preoperative evaluation of these patients includes a complete medical history, psychological history, nutritional assessment, physical examination, and investigations to assess surgical risk for metabolic surgery (endocrine, metabolic, nutritional, and psychological assessments). In 2008, American Association of Clinical Endocrinologists (AACE), TOS, and American Society for Metabolic and Bariatric Surgery (ASMBS) published clinical practice guidelines (CPG) for perioperative nutritional, metabolic, and nonsurgical support of the bariatric surgery patients,[8] which was recently updated in 2013.[9] Patients should have a comprehensive preoperative assessment of all comorbid conditions. For patients with diabetes, they should be counseled regarding frequent postoperative monitoring of glycemic control, diabetic complications

Table 1	
Indications and contraindications for surgery to treat type 2 diabetes	
Indication (BMI depends on patients' ancestry; Asians: BMI should be reduced by 2.5 kg/m²)	Recommended in: • T2D patients with class III obesity (BMI ≥40 kg/m²); regardless of glycemic control or complexity of glucose-lowering regimes • T2D patients with class II obesity (BMI 35–39.9 kg/m²) with inadequate glycemic control despite lifestyle and optimal medical treatment (either oral or injectable medications including insulin) Considered in: • T2D patients with class I obesity (BMI 30–34.9 kg/m²) with inadequate glycemic control despite optimal medical treatment (oral or injectable medications, including insulin) • The patient must be psychiatrically stable
Contraindication	Relative contraindication • High risk of surgical complication due to poor health • Inability or unwillingness to change lifestyle postoperatively • Uncommitted to long-term follow-up and nutritional supplementation postoperatively • Addicted to drugs or alcohol • Psychologically unstable

(diabetic ketoacidosis or hypoglycemia), the likelihood of diabetes remission, and complementary medical therapy.

The choice of the metabolic procedure is based on the risk-to-benefit-ratio evaluation for each patient. Long-term postoperative complications of surgery versus effectiveness of glycemic and cardiovascular risk should be discussed with each patient as part of informed consent. Currently, 4 procedures constitute most bariatric operations globally: SG, RYGB, LAGB, and BPD + DS (**Fig. 1**).

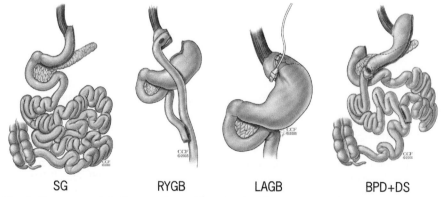

SG   RYGB   LAGB   BPD+DS

Fig. 1. Common metabolic procedures. (*Reprinted with* permission, Cleveland Clinic Center for Medical Art & Photography © 2006-2016. All Rights Reserved.)

Table 2
Patient preparation (in operation room)

Positioning	• Supine position with the feet together on a footboard • Heavy tape is used to secure the patient's legs to the bed above and below the knees to prevent the knees from bending when the patient is in full reverse Trendelenburg position
Prophylactic antibiotics	• First-generation cephalosporin or an appropriate alternative in patients allergic to penicillin
VTE prophylaxis	• Intermittent pneumatic compression devices are applied to lower limb • Intraoperative chemoprophylaxis

TECHNIQUE OF THE PROCEDURES

Patient preparation in the operating room is summarized in **Table 2**. The position of the operating surgeon and the assistant is as shown in **Figs. 2**, and **3** shows the port placement for all the bariatric procedures in the authors' center.

Approach

Liver retraction

A 5-mm liver retractor (Snowden-Pencer, Tucker, GA, USA) is placed through the right lateral port and anchored to the bed with a self-retaining device. A Nathanson liver

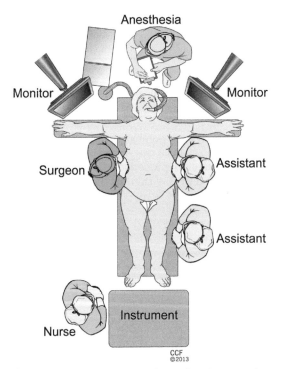

Fig. 2. Positioning for laparoscopic surgery. In the authors' center, the operating surgeon stands on the patient's right side and the assistant stands on the left for all bariatric procedures. Monitors are placed on both sides of the table over the patient's shoulder. (*Reprinted with* permission, Cleveland Clinic Center for Medical Art & Photography © 2006-2016. All Rights Reserved.)

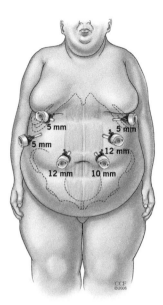

Fig. 3. Port placement. Pneumoperitoneum: Established with a Veress needle through a left upper quadrant incision. Visual access to the peritoneal cavity: Use a 5-mm optical viewing trocar, and the remaining 5 ports are placed under direct vision. Ports placement for all bariatric procedures is as shown. If there are severe adhesions to the abdominal wall from a prior laparotomy, an additional 5-mm trocar is placed in the left lower quadrant to create an adequate working space for the remaining ports. (*Reprinted with permission, Cleveland Clinic Center for Medical Art & Photography © 2006-2016. All Rights Reserved.*)

retractor can also be used in the subxiphoid position and, for larger patients with extremely big or floppy left hepatic lobes, both retractor systems can be used simultaneously to achieve adequate exposure of the gastroesophageal junction.

Operative Procedures

Sleeve gastrectomy

- Mobilize the omentum at stomach's greater curvature from the angle of His all the way down to the pylorus using the ultrasonic dissector device.
- Create stomach tube (**Fig. 4**A).
  - Once the stomach is fully mobilized, apply a 60 mm load stapler approximately 3 cm to the pylorus, parallel to the lesser curvature. An endoscope is passed down along the lesser curvature of the stomach and into the pylorus. Continue to fire 60 mm load staplers parallel to the endoscope up toward the angle of His.
- Oversewn stapler lines
  - The long stapler lines are oversewn with running a 2-0 absorbable suture in a Lembert fashion all the way down to the pylorus. Alternatively, some surgeons will reinforce the staple line with a synthetic buttressing material or provide no additional reinforcement. **Fig. 4**B shows the final anastomotic arrangement after SG.
- Leak test
  - With the scope in place, insufflation of stomach is performed to test for air leaks and narrowing.
- Schauer's cap

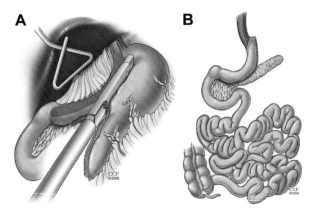

Fig. 4. The laparoscopic SG. (*A*) Creating a narrow gastric tube over a bougie or endoscope using a linear cutting stapler to excise the stomach body and fundus. (*B*) The final anatomic arrangement after a SG. (*Reprinted with* permission, Cleveland Clinic Center for Medical Art & Photography © 2006-2016. All Rights Reserved.)

- An omental patch is placed over the anastomosis and secured with 2-0 nonabsorbable suture.
- Liver biopsy
  - A core needle liver biopsy using an 18-G needle is performed routinely as part of every bariatric procedure to document the severity of nonalcoholic fatty liver disease (NAFLD).
- Drain (optional)
  - A round Jackson-Pratt (JP) drain is placed alongside the staple/suture line and brought out through the right upper quadrant port site.
- Specimen retrieval (SG)
  - A remnant stomach specimen is removed using a sterile bag.
- Port closure
  - Close fascia at the 12-mm port sites with absorbable suture using a suture-passer.
- Skin closure
  - All instruments and trocars are removed. The abdomen is deflated.
  - Skin incisions are closed with subcuticular 4-0 absorbable suture.
- Sterile dressings are applied.

Adjustable gastric band

- Gastrohepatic ligament window creation
  - After adequate exposure of the gastroesophageal junction, the peritoneum overlying the angle of His is divided with a Harmonic scalpel. The pars flaccida is opened, and the base of the right crus is identified.
- Before the gastric band is placed, the band, its tubing, and port are tested for no leak and functioning well.
- Band placement (**Fig. 5**A)
  - An opening is created at the base of the right crus, and the articulating band passer device is passed through the retrogastric tunnel to the left side and held in place. The band is then placed in the abdominal cavity and attached to the band passer. Once the band is placed well, it is then locked around the upper portion of the stomach.

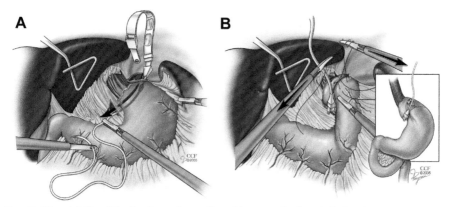

Fig. 5. The LAGB. (*A*) Passing the adjustable gastric band behind the posterior stomach wall through a window in the gastrohepatic ligament (pars-flaccida technique). (*B*) Placing a few loose, simple interrupted plication sutures over the band anteriorly to reduce risk of band slippage and stomach herniation. (*Reprinted with permission, Cleveland Clinic Center for Medical Art & Photography © 2006-2016. All Rights Reserved.*)

- Stomach-band stay suture (see **Fig. 5**B)
  - Two gastrogastric plication sutures are placed using 0 silk sutures, and the removable attachment of the band is then removed through the 15-mm trocar site.
- Port placement
  - A subcutaneous pocket is created at the right paramedian 15-mm trocar site. The band tubing is brought out through that opening. The fascia is cleared inferior and lateral to the exit site, and the tubing is pushed into the abdomen without any tension. The port applicator is used to secure the port to the fascia so it is held in good position.
- Final laparoscopic inspection to look for the band position; no kinks or twisting of the tubing.

Roux-en-Y gastric bypass
Roux-en-Y gastric bypass is one of the commonest metabolic surgery performed with excellent weight loss and metabolic disease improvement (**Fig. 6**).

Other Gastrojejunal Anastomosis Options

The gastrojejunal anastomosis has various techniques: using the linear stapler (mentioned earlier), circular stapler, or hand-sewn. Currently, the authors performed hand-sewn gastrojejunostomy most often.

Completely hand-sewn anastomoses are used by many open bariatric surgeons and some laparoscopic bariatric surgeons. This technique has the advantages of using less specialized equipment and eliminating the need to enlarge a port site for the circular stapler. The hand-sewn technique, though, requires considerable skill to complete at an appropriate time. After the gastric pouch is created, a 2-layer 10- to 12-mm anastomosis is created over a calibration tube with 3-0 absorbable sutures.

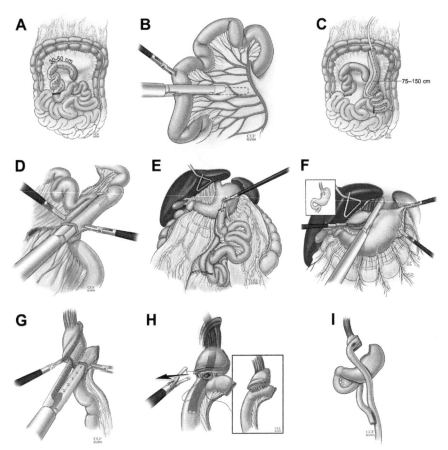

Fig. 6. The steps in the authors' laparoscopic RYGB approach. (*A*) Once pneumoperitoneum is created and ports are inserted as mentioned in the text, the transverse colon and omentum are reflected superiorly to the upper abdomen and the ligament of Treitz is identified. The assistant should hold the mesocolon upward with a grasper to maintain adequate exposure during creation of the JJ. (*B*) "C" configuration of the proximal jejunum toward the camera helps in the orientation of the proximal and distal segments. The jejunum is divided 50 cm from the ligament of Treitz with a 60-mm load stapler. (*C*) The Roux limb is measured distally from the marked stitch for a distance of 150 cm. (*D*) JJ anastomosis. The bowel should be straightened (not stretched) against a rigid measuring device such as a marked grasper to determine the proper Roux limb length. Once the appropriate length is measured, a suture is placed to approximate the biliopancreatic limb and the Roux limb side by side. With the assistant holding upward on the stay suture, small adjacent enterotomies are made with an ultrasonic dissector and a 60-mm load stapler is applied, to create an end-to-side JJ anastomosis. The enterotomy site is closed with another 60-mm load stapler. A supportive stitch is placed at the far angle of the enteroenterostomy using 2-0 nonabsorbable suture. An antiobstruction stitch is placed to approximate the Roux limb to the biliopancreatic limb with 2-0 nonabsorbable suture. The residual mesenteric defect is closed with running 2-0 nonabsorbable suture. (*E*) The patient is then placed in the reverse Trendelenburg position. The omentum is split down the middle using an ultrasonic dissector to reduce tension. The Roux limb is then advanced to an antecolic antegastric fashion up toward the stomach. (*F*) Gastric pouch creation. A window is created in the gastrohepatic ligament with an ultrasonic dissector. After the anesthesiologist removes all intragastric devices, a 60-mm load stapler is fired across the

Gastric Pouch Ring Placement

If the patient has BMI > 50 kg/m2, an additional gastric pouch ring (**Fig. 7**) can be placed to prevent gastric pouch dilatation and weight regain. We selectively place a silicone ring around the gastric pouch for super obese patients to provide additional long-term restriction. A 10-cm-long 8-Fr silicone tube (2 mm wide) is used in these cases. The authors place a silk suture 1.75 cm from each end of the silastic tubing, which leaves 6.5 cm of the band to encircle the pouch when it is placed. After the GJ has been completed, a small opening is created in the peritoneum overlying the base of the right crus, and an instrument is passed using the pars flaccida technique. The silicone tubing is grasped and pulled into place around the upper pouch with the endoscope still in place through the GJ. The surgeon and the assistant grab the ends

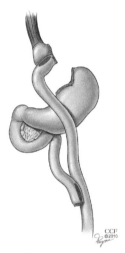

Fig. 7. Gastric pouch ring placement. The authors selectively place a silicone ring around the gastric pouch for superobese patients to provide additional long-term restriction. (*Reprinted with* permission, Cleveland Clinic Center for Medical Art & Photography © 2006-2016. All Rights Reserved.)

mesentery of the lesser curvature, and 3 × 60-mm load staplers are fired across the gastric cardia to create a 15-mL gastric pouch. Staple lines are examined on both sides and hemostasis is secured. (*G*) The end of the Roux limb is sutured to the posterior aspect of the gastric pouch using 2-0 nonabsorbable suture. Enterotomies are made in the gastric pouch and in the Roux limb with an ultrasonic dissector. A 60-mm load stapler is inserted approximately 2 cm into the pouch and applied to create a stapled end-to-end gastrojejunostomy (GJ). Alternatively, a circular stapler can be used or a hand-sewn technique to create the GJ (see later discussion). (*H*) GJ anastomosis flexible endoscopy is performed. The scope is passed down the esophagus through the anastomosis and into the Roux limb. The enterotomy is closed with the endoscope in place as a stent. It is closed in running fashion to bring in both corners and tie in the middle using 2-0 nonabsorbable suture. A second anterior layer with 2-0 nonabsorbable suture has approximated the Roux limb and encompassed the gastric pouch staple line beginning from the greater curvature side to the lesser curvature side. (*I*) The final anatomic RYGB. (*Reprinted with* permission, Cleveland Clinic Center for Medical Art & Photography © 2006-2016. All Rights Reserved.)

of the tubing and bring the 2 sutures together over the anterior pouch. Clips are placed across the overlapping tubing to hold the ring in place, and the sutures are then tied together. The ring should be approximately 2 or 3 cm above the GJ, and this can be confirmed endoscopically.

Biliopancreatic diversion/duodenal switch

Biliopancreatic diversion/duodenal switch (BPD/DS) is not commonly performed now days. However, BPD/DS has the best long term outcome among all the metabolic procedures in term of weight loss and resolution of metabolic disease (**Fig. 8**).

- Jejunojejunostomy (JJ) creation
  - The distal ileum 100 to 150 cm from the cecum is measured and marked with a stitch. Then, an additional 150 cm proximal is measured, and that is marked with a stitch. Then, the bowel is divided at that point with an application of a 60-mm load stapler. The proximal end of that cut bowel is then connected in an end-to-side fashion 100 to 150 cm from the cecum. A nonabsorbable stay suture of 2-0 is applied. Enterotomies are made in each of the bowel limbs. An end-to-end anastomosis is performed using the 60-mm load stapler. The mesenteric defect is closed with running 2-0 nonabsorbable suture.
- Stomach tube creation
  - The stomach is then sleeved as in SG.
- Duodenal ileostomy
  - The duodenum is mobilized approximately 3 to 4 cm from the pylorus. The duodenum is transected using a 60-mm load stapler, and the duodenal stump is oversewn with a running 2-0 nonabsorbable suture.

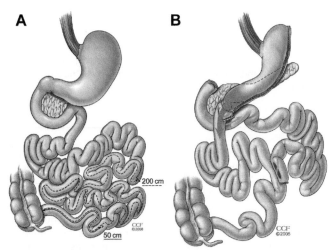

Fig. 8. The biliopancreatic diversion. (*A*) Sites of first and second small bowel transection points are marked. The 50-cm and 200-cm marks shown are for the standard (Scopinaro) BPD. (*B*) For the BPD + DS, small bowel transected at 100 cm and 250 cm from the ilealcecal valve, respectively (250-cm alimentary limb and 100-cm common channel). (*Reprinted with permission, Cleveland Clinic Center for Medical Art & Photography © 2006-2016. All Rights Reserved.*)

○ The cut end of the ileum is then attached to the proximal duodenal stump in an end-to-side fashion with a posterior layer of running 2-0 nonabsorbable suture. Enterotomies are made on each side of the bowel with an ultrasonic dissector. The posterior layer is closed with 2-0 absorbable suture. The anterior layer is completed with 2-0 absorbable suture with the endoscope through the anastomosis. Then, a final anastomosis is completed by a running 2-0 absorbable suture.

Complications and Management

The complications of metabolic surgery are multifactorial and can arise from chronic obesity and comorbidities or related to the surgical procedures. Men, smokers, older age, higher BMI, the presence of multiple comorbidities, or prior revisional surgeries have a higher risk of postoperative complications.[10]

Postoperative complications can be divided into general (**Table 3**) or procedure-related complications (**Table 4**). The general complications usually occur during the immediate or early postoperative period. General complications include infection, hemorrhage, and venous thromboembolism (VTE). Infection can be either intra-abdominal infection (abscess collection, peritonitis), catheter-related infection, pneumonia, and surgical site infections. Preventive

Table 3	
General complications of metabolic surgery and frequency	
	Frequency (%)
Sepsis from anastomotic leak	0.1–5.6
Hemorrhage	1–4
Cardiopulmonary events	<1
VTE	0.34
Death	0.1–0.3
AGB-related complications:	
Band slippage	15
Leakage	2–5
Erosion	1–2
Bypass procedures–related complications:	
Anastomotic stricture	1–5
Marginal ulcers	1–5
Bowel obstructions	0.5–2
Nutrition deficiencies from:	
RYGB	
Iron deficiency	45–52
Vitamin B_{12} deficiency	8–37
Calcium deficiency	10
Vitamin D deficiency	51
BPD + DS	
Fat-soluble vitamin deficiencies (A, D, E, K)	1–5
Protein malnutrition	1–5

Table 4
Procedure-related complications and the management

Complication	Clinical Presentation	Diagnostic Investigation	Management
Gastrointestinal leak (SG, RYGB, BPD ± DS)	• Tachycardia, hypotension, tachypnoeic, fever, abdominal ± chest pain	• Upper gastrointestinal (UGI) studies or computed tomographic (CT) abdomen	• Stable patient with contained leak • Percutaneous drainage and antibiotics • Surgical intervention (repair if feasible, irrigation, drainage, and feeding tube)
Hemorrhage (SG, RYGB, BPD ± DS)	• Tachycardia, hypotension, bloody drain, drop in hemoglobin	• Stable patient: upper endoscopy • Unstable patient: surgical intervention	• Stable patient: endoscopic intervention • Unstable patient: surgical intervention (stapler line oversewn, clips, hemostatic agents)
Gastric remnant dilatation (RYGB)	• Hiccups, bloating, sepsis	• Abdominal radiograph	• Decompression (percutaneous or surgical)
Small bowel obstruction (RYGB, BPD ± DS)	• Intermittent colicky abdominal pain with distension, nausea, vomiting	• CT abdomen • Small bowel series • Diagnostic laparoscopy	• Surgical intervention
Stricture/anastomotic stenosis (SG, RYGB, BPD ± DS)	• Present 2 wk to 6 mo postoperatively with vomiting or food intolerance	• Upper endoscopy	• Endoscopic balloon dilatation
Marginal ulcer (RYGB)	• Nausea, vomiting, abdominal pain, UGI bleeding	• Upper endoscopy • UGI contrast study	• Avoid NSAIDs, smoking • Proton pump inhibitor • Sucralfate therapy
Gastrogastric fistula (RYGB)	• Nausea, vomiting, epigastric pain, bleeding in cases with the marginal ulcer, failure to lose weight or weight regain	• UGI contrast study • CT abdomen • Upper endoscopy (can be missed in small fistula)	• Proton pump inhibitor (for remnant stomach) • Sucralfate (for gastric pouch) • Surgical intervention (if conservative management fails or patients unable to lose weight)

Reflux (SG, AGB)	• Nausea, vomiting	• Upper endoscopy	• Proton pump inhibitor • Surgical intervention if worsening evidence of gastroesophageal reflux grade C or D
Nutritional deficiencies (SG, RYGB, BPD ± DS)	• Depends on vitamin or mineral deficiency • Anemia symptoms	• Blood investigation on the vitamin and mineral levels • Hemoglobin, iron, and B12 levels	• Routine follow-up with multivitamin supplements and replacement of the deficiencies (vitamin or mineral) • Iron or B12 replacement • Pack cell transfusion in severe cases
Gallstone (RYGB, BPD ± DS)	• Biliary colic or acute cholecystitis symptoms	• Ultrasound abdomen	• Ursodiol 6 mo postoperative to reduce risk of gallstone formation • Cholecystectomy
Weight regain or failure to lose weight (SG, AGB, RYGB, BPD ± DS)	• Unsatisfactory weight changes • Recurrence of comorbidity-related symptoms	• CT abdomen • Small bowel series • Diagnostic laparoscopy	• Bariatric surgeon re-evaluation • Medical weight management • Surgical revision as necessary
Specific for AGB complications			
Band erosion	• Nausea, vomiting, or bleeding	• Upper endoscopy	• Removal of gastric band (endoscopy or laparoscopy)
Band slippage ± gastric prolapse	• Nausea, vomiting	• Abdominal radiograph	• Laparoscopic removal of gastric band
Port or tube-related complication	• Depends on the cause (migration, kinking, leak, or infection)	• Abdominal radiograph	• Surgical intervention

Abbreviation: NSAIDs, nonsteroidal anti-inflammatory drugs.

management includes prophylactic antibiotic usage, such as cephalosporin, aggressive lung physiotherapy, and early ambulation. Hemorrhage can either be intra-abdominal or upper gastrointestinal hemorrhage. It can occur as immediate or early postoperatively at the stapler line, anastomotic site, or surgical incision sites. The usage of anticoagulant has a slight increase in bleeding tendencies in these patients.

VTE is the commonest cause of postoperative mortality after bariatric surgery, and 80% of VTE occurs after the patient is discharged from the hospital. The overall 30-day incidence of post-discharge VTE was 0.29%, and the mortality caused by the VTE post-discharge increased by 28-fold.[11] Bariatric patients with congestive heart failure, paraplegia, dyspnea at rest, and who underwent reoperation are associated with higher risk of post-discharge VTE incidence. Therefore, extended chemoprophylaxis in this high-risk group would be beneficial to reduce the incidence of post-discharge VTE. ASMBS has published the general recommendations for VTE prophylaxis for patients undergoing bariatric surgery: early ambulation and the use of mechanical VTE prophylaxis such as sequential compression devices or elastic compression stockings, and chemoprophylaxis. However, there is no consensus regarding type, dosage, and duration of chemoprophylaxis.[12]

POSTOPERATIVE CARE

Postoperative care should be managed by a multidisciplinary team (surgeon, endocrinologist/diabetologist, nutritionist, and nurses with diabetic expertise). The postoperative care after metabolic surgery is based on the DSS-II joint statement guidelines[7] and the CPG in perioperative nutritional, metabolic, and nonsurgical support of the bariatric surgery patients by the AACE/TOS/ASMBS.[9] **Tables 5** and **6** outlined the postoperative care.

Table 5 Early postoperative care	
Cardiopulmonary care	• High risk of myocardial infarction: at least 24 h telemetry monitoring • Pulmonary toilet, incentive spirometry • Early continuous positive airway pressure if required • Deep vein thrombosis prophylaxis, encourage ambulation • If unstable: consider leak or pulmonary embolism
Hydration	• Maintain adequate hydration (usually 1.5 L per day orally)
Healthy eating education	• Protocol-derived stage meal progression by nutritionist
Monitoring	• Blood glucose levels • Watch out for hypoglycemic symptoms
Pressure sore prevention	• Early ambulation • Adequate padding at pressure points • If suspected rhabdomyolysis: check for creatine kinase level
Medications	• 1- 2 adult multivitamin-mineral supplements containing iron, 1200 to 1500 mg/d of calcium, and a vitamin B-complex preparation • Anti-diabetes medications adjustment based on glycemic control

Table 6 Follow-up care	
Follow-up visit (depends on the condition of patients and type of metabolic surgery)	• Nutritional, diabetes, and surgical evaluation at least every 6 mo for the first 2 y postoperatively and annually
Monitoring	• HbA1c every 3 mo first 2 y postoperatively • Weight-loss trend • Nutritional assessment (long term) ○ Micronutrient monitoring, nutritional supplementation, and support • Psychological assessment (if support group needed) • Evaluate for postoperative complications • Physical activity monitoring (>150 min of aerobic activity per week)
Evaluation and adjustment of T2D	• For first 6 mo, careful evaluation of glycemic control and anti-diabetes medications • If plasma glucose level rapidly reaching normal level in the early postoperative period, careful adjustment of medical therapy is necessary to prevent hypoglycemia. Choose low-risk hypoglycemia drugs (metformin or other oral hypoglycemic agents) • After the initial 6 mo, anti-diabetes medications should be tapered based on documented HbA1c levels
Evaluation and adjustment	• Adjust treatment of other cardiovascular risks (hypertension and dyslipidemia medications based on laboratory results)
Avoid	• Nonsteroidal anti-inflammatory drugs, steroids, smoking to prevent peptic ulcers
Prophylactic medication	• For gout and gallstone in appropriate patients

OUTCOMES

Significant evidence suggests that metabolic surgery results in durable weight loss and improvement in obesity-related comorbidities (**Fig. 9**).

Weight Loss

Bariatric surgery is the only therapeutic intervention in severely obese patients that is proven to produce clinically significant and sustained weight loss for more than 5 years. Typically, bariatric surgery results in a 20- to 40-kg weight loss and a 10- to 15-kg/m^2 BMI reduction, but the weight loss varies between the bariatric procedures. In the SOS trial[13] evaluating long-term effects of bariatric surgery compared with nonsurgical weight management in obese patients (BMI >34 kg/m^2) at 10, 15, and 20 years, the mean changes in body weight were −17%, −16%, and −18% in bariatric surgical groups as compared with control group; 1%, −1%, and −1%, respectively. The mean weight loss (kg) after 10 years for gastric banding, vertical banded gastroplasty, and gastric bypass was 14 kg, 16 kg, and 25 kg. A meta-analysis conducted by Buchwald and colleagues[14] showed that overall weight loss and percentage of excess weight loss after bariatric surgery were 38.5 kg and 55.9%, respectively.

Type 2 Diabetes Remission and Improvement

Metabolic surgery has shown significant resolution in T2D in both observational and randomized controlled trials (RCTs). A recent systemic review involving 73 studies

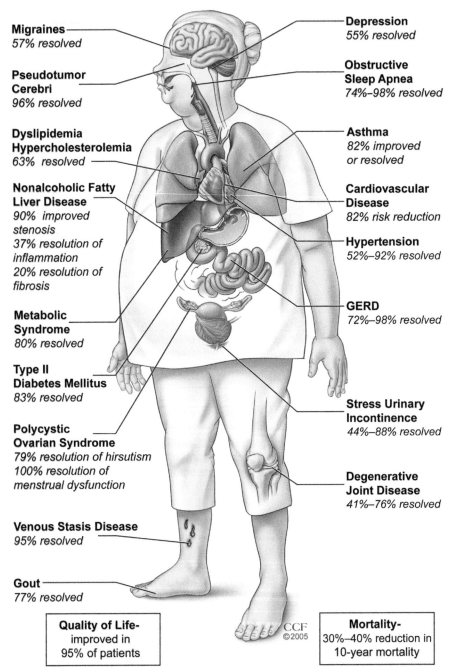

Migraines
57% resolved

Pseudotumor Cerebri
96% resolved

Dyslipidemia Hypercholesterolemia
63% resolved

Nonalcoholic Fatty Liver Disease
90% improved stenosis
37% resolution of inflammation
20% resolution of fibrosis

Metabolic Syndrome
80% resolved

Type II Diabetes Mellitus
83% resolved

Polycystic Ovarian Syndrome
79% resolution of hirsutism
100% resolution of menstrual dysfunction

Venous Stasis Disease
95% resolved

Gout
77% resolved

Depression
55% resolved

Obstructive Sleep Apnea
74%–98% resolved

Asthma
82% improved or resolved

Cardiovascular Disease
82% risk reduction

Hypertension
52%–92% resolved

GERD
72%–98% resolved

Stress Urinary Incontinence
44%–88% resolved

Degenerative Joint Disease
41%–76% resolved

Quality of Life- improved in 95% of patients

CCF
©2005

Mortality- 30%–40% reduction in 10-year mortality

Fig. 9. Outcome of metabolic surgery in obesity-related comorbidities. GERD, gastroesophageal reflux disease. (*Reprinted with* permission, Cleveland Clinic Center for Medical Art & Photography © 2006-2016. All Rights Reserved.)

with 19,543 patients at a mean follow-up of 57.8 months showed a remission/improvement for T2D of 73%.[15] Buchwald and colleagues[14] in their meta-analysis on the impact of bariatric surgery in T2D patients (621 studies, 135,246 patients) showed a 78% complete resolution rate, and 87% of diabetic patients had either improvement or resolution of T2D. BPD ± DS has the best T2D resolution (95.9%), followed by gastric bypass (70.9%) and gastric band (58.3%) at 2-year follow-up. The 3-year outcome of the STAMPEDE trial showed that bariatric surgery versus intensive medical therapy had a significant number of T2D patients with glycated hemoglobin level less than or equal to 6.0%; 38% in gastric bypass group, 24% in SG group, and 5% in the medical-therapy group ($P<.001$).[16] Recently, Schauer and colleagues[1] reviewed 11 RCTs (involving 794 T2D patients with a follow-up period of 6 months to 5 years), comparing metabolic surgery with medical treatment. All the RCTs showed significant outcome T2D resolution in the surgery group as compared with the medical treatment ($P<.05$) except one study. Ding and colleagues[17] showed diabetic remission for LAGB and medical treatment was 33% and 23%, respectively ($P = .46$). Panunzi and colleagues[18] showed in a meta-analysis that diabetes resolution was 89% after biliopancreatic diversion, 77% after RYGB, 62% after gastric banding, and 60% after SG.

With respect to reduction in long-term complications of diabetes, Schauer and colleagues[16] in the STAMPEDE trial showed modest improvement in albuminuria 3 years after surgery, but there was no improvement or worsening of retinopathy. In the SOS trial,[19,20] bariatric surgery had a 50% reduction in microvascular complications of diabetes, significant improvement of glycemic control, and cardiovascular risk factors compared with the medical treatment group. Among the 11 RCTs comparing surgery to medical treatment of T2D, none had sufficient duration of follow-up or were powered sufficiently to detect differences in macrovascular or microvascular events between surgical and control patients.[1]

Cardiovascular Risk Reduction

Metabolic surgery has also shown improvement in obesity-related comorbidities such as hypertension, hyperlipidemia, and cardiovascular disease (CVD). The SOS trial[13] showed significantly decreased rates of myocardial infarction, stroke, cardiovascular mortality, cancer mortality, and all-cause mortality after bariatric surgery. Bolen and colleagues[21] at 5 years showed 53% resolution or improvement in hypercholesterolemia, and Sugerman and colleagues[22] showed 66% resolution or improvement in hypertension in 7 years. A systemic review of cardiovascular outcomes after bariatric surgery showed evidence of left ventricular hypertrophy regression and improvement of diastolic function after bariatric surgery.[15] There were improvement and resolution of hyperlipidemia (65%), hypertension (63%), and all-cause mortality as compared with the nonsurgical group.

Current Controversies and Future Considerations

Cirrhosis improvement after metabolic surgery
Nonalcoholic steatohepatitis (NASH) is a subset of NAFLD, with a prevalence of 25% to 55% in patients with obesity, and up to 15% to 20% of proven NASH will progress into cirrhosis.[23,24] NASH is a histologic diagnosis characterized by steatosis in greater than 5% of hepatocytes, hepatocellular ballooning, and lobular inflammation.[25] Studies have shown a significant improvement in liver function studies and also histologic changes in NASH patients after bariatric surgery.[26–28] A systemic review conducted by Rabl and Campos[29] (involving 20 studies, 1502 patients) showed histologic improvement in NASH after bariatric surgery irrespective of bariatric procedures. Patients with NASH and advanced liver disease also showed improvement in all

histologic components of cirrhosis, including steatosis, inflammation, and fibrosis after bariatric procedures, especially RYGB.

In patients with frank cirrhosis, the outcome of bariatric surgery and the histologic changes are limited. In most cases, cirrhosis in bariatric patients is diagnosed intraoperatively, with an incidence of approximately 2%.[30] Bariatric surgery was thought to be contraindicated in these high-risk patients due to the potential risk of cirrhosis-related complications and mortality. However, a recent systemic review has shown that bariatric surgery in Child-Pugh A cirrhotic patients is relatively safe with major morbidities and mortalities much lower than expected: 21.3% and 1.6%, respectively. The delayed mortality (>30 days) was 2.5%, and postsurgical liver decompensation was only 6.6%.[31] However, outcomes in more advanced cirrhotic patients (Child-Pugh B and C) are still not well documented.

Metabolic surgery in patients with diabetes and mild obesity (body mass index 30–34)
Recent studies have shown that metabolic surgery in patients with mild obesity (BMI 30–34) can result in improvement and remission of diabetes just as effectively as patients with BMI greater than or equal to 35. A meta-analysis on predictors of diabetes remission was conducted on 94,579 bariatric surgical patients with BMI less than 35 kg/m^2 and BMI greater than 35 kg/m^2. The study showed that diabetic remission in patients with BMI less than 35 kg/m^2 was 72% and patients with BMI greater than 35 kg/m^2 was 71%. Diabetic remission in BPD, RYGB, adjustable gastric band (AGB), and SG was 89%, 77%, 62%, and 60%, respectively.[18] The only predictor of diabetic remission in this study was waist circumference but not BMI, suggesting that the arbitrary exclusion of patients with BMI less than 35 is not scientifically valid.[18] The STAMPEDE RCT study demonstrated that patients with BMI 27 to 34 achieved similar improvements in hemoglobin A1c (HbA1c) compared with patients with BMI greater than 35.[16] Furthermore, most of the 11 RCTs comparing metabolic surgery to medical treatment of T2D included patients with BMI less than 35.[1] Collectively, these studies confirmed equivalent benefit for patients with mild obesity compared with the severely obese, and there appeared to be no increased risk of excessive weight loss or nutritional complications in this lower BMI group. Consequently, the new international guidelines for metabolic surgery do recommend consideration of surgery for patients with T2D and BMI 30 to 34 who are not well controlled on diabetes medications.[7] For patients at higher risk of diabetes complications such as people from Asian descent, the BMI threshold was reduced to a BMI of 27.5. This new concept of surgery for diabetes and mild obesity is a significant departure from the long-held belief that patients must have severe obesity to justify surgery.

Further research is needed for the optimal time to intervene patients for metabolic surgery, selection of metabolic procedures, and specific criteria for metabolic surgery in T2D patients besides BMI alone. Long-term RCT studies on CVD, mortality, and other outcomes in these patients and the adolescent population are also needed.

SUMMARY

Outcomes of bariatric and metabolic surgery have steadily improved over the last half-century especially after the advent of minimally invasive laparoscopic techniques. The most common procedures include SG, gastric bypass, gastric banding, and duodenal switch with SG and gastric bypass contriving more than 80% of all weight-loss procedures. Today, more than 95% of all bariatric operations are performed with laparoscopic surgery. Morbidities (5%) and mortalities (0.1%–0.3%) of bariatric surgery are very similar to that of "low-risk" procedures such as laparoscopic cholecystectomy and hysterectomy. The most important complications include bleeding, VTE, leaks, bowel obstruction, ulcers, and strictures. Long-term nutritional deficiencies are generally preventable with vitamin and nutrient supplementation, although mild anemia is common (10%–20%). Long-term weight loss varies depending on the procedure and patient factors such as preoperative BMI but averages around 15% to 25% 5 years and beyond. Most comorbidities, such as T2D, hypertension, dyslipidemia, sleep apnea, arthritis, gastroesophageal reflux disease, and NAFLD, improve or resolve after surgery. Diabetes responds very well to metabolic surgery particularly in the early stages when remission is possible. Some longitudinal cohort studies suggest mortality reduction with bariatric surgery. Given the current epidemiologic trends in obesity together with improving outcomes of surgery, metabolic surgery is likely to play a more prominent role in the management of obesity and diabetes in the immediate future.

REFERENCES

1. Schauer PR, Mingrone G, Ikramuddin S, et al. Clinical outcomes of metabolic surgery: efficacy of glycemic control, weight loss, and remission of diabetes. Diabetes Care 2016;39(6):902–11.

2. Brethauer SA, Chand B, Schauer PR. Risks and benefits of bariatric surgery: current evidence. Cleveland Clinic J Med 2006;73(11):993.

3. Ponce J, DeMaria EJ, Nguyen NT, et al. American Society for Metabolic and Bariatric Surgery estimation of bariatric surgery procedures in 2015 and surgeon workforce in the United States. Surg Obes Relat Dis 2016;12(9):1637–9.

4. NIH conference. Gastrointestinal surgery for severe obesity. Consensus Development Conference Panel. Ann Intern Med 1991;115:956–61.

5. Jensen MD, Ryan DH, Apovian CM, et al, American College of Cardiology/American Heart Association Task Force on Practice Guidelines, The Obesity Society. 2013 AHA/ACC/TOS guideline for the management of overweight and obesity in adults: a report of the American College of Cardiology/American Heart Association Task Force on Practice Guidelines and The Obesity Society. J Am Coll Cardiol 2014;63: 2985–3023 [Erratum appears in J Am Coll Cardiol 2014;63:3029–30].

6. Livingston EH. Inadequacy of BMI as an indicator for bariatric surgery. JAMA 2012;307:88–9.

7. Rubino F, Nathan DM, Eckel RH, et al. Metabolic surgery in the treatment algorithm for type 2 diabetes: a joint statement by international diabetes organizations. Diabetes care 2016;39(6):861–77.

8. Mechanick JI, Kushner RF, Sugerman HJ, et al. American Association of Clinical Endocrinologists, The Obesity Society, and American Society for Metabolic & Bariatric Surgery Medical Guidelines for Clinical Practice for the perioperative nutritional, metabolic, and nonsurgical support of the bariatric surgery patient. Surg Obes Relat Dis 2008;4(5):S109–84.

9. Mechanick JI, Youdim A, Jones DB, et al. Clinical practice guidelines for the perioperative nutritional, metabolic, and nonsurgical support of the bariatric surgery patient—2013 update: Cosponsored by American Association of Clinical Endocrinologists, The Obesity Society, and American Society for Metabolic & Bariatric Surgery. Obesity 2013;21(S1):S1–27.

10. Longitudinal Assessment of Bariatric Surgery (LABS) Consortium, Flum DR, Belle SH, King WC, et al. Perioperative safety in the longitudinal assessment of bariatric surgery. N Engl J Med 2009;2009(361):445–54.

11. Aminian A, Andalib A, Khorgami Z, et al. Who should get extended thromboprophylaxis after bariatric surgery? A risk assessment tool to guide indications for post-discharge pharmacoprophylaxis. Ann Surg 2017;265(1):143–50.

12. The American Society for Metabolic and Bariatric Surgery Clinical Issues Committee. ASMBS updated position statement on prophylactic measures to reduce the risk of venous thromboembolism in bariatric surgery patients. Surg Obes Relat Dis 2013;9(4):493–7.

13. Sjöström L, Peltonen M, Jacobson P, et al. Bariatric surgery and long-term cardiovascular events. JAMA 2012;307(1):56–65.

14. Buchwald H, Estok R, Fahrbach K, et al. Weight and type 2 diabetes after bariatric surgery: systematic review and meta-analysis. Am J Med 2009;122(3):248–56.

15. Vest AR, Heneghan HM, Agarwal S, et al. Bariatric surgery and cardiovascular outcomes: a systematic review. Heart 2012;98:1763–77.

16. Schauer PR, Bhatt DL, Kirwan JP, et al, STAMPEDE Investigators. Bariatric surgery versus intensive medical therapy for diabetes–3-year outcomes. N Engl J Med 2014;370:2002–13.

17. Ding SA, Simonson DC, Wewalka M, et al. Adjustable gastric band surgery or medical management in patients with type 2 diabetes: a randomized clinical trial. J Clin Endocrinol Metab 2015;100(7):2546–56.

18. Panunzi S, De Gaetano A, Carnicelli A, et al. Predictors of remission of diabetes mellitus in severely obese individuals undergoing bariatric surgery: do BMI or procedure choice matter? A meta-analysis. Ann Surg 2015;261(3):459–67.

19. Sjöström L, Peltonen M, Jacobson P, et al. Association of bariatric surgery with long-term remission of type 2 diabetes and with microvascular and macrovascular complications. JAMA 2014;311(22):2297–304.

20. Sjöström L, Lindroos AK, Peltonen M, et al. Lifestyle, diabetes, and cardiovascular risk factors 10 years after bariatric surgery. Engl J Med 2004;351(26):2683–93.

21. Bolen SD, Chang HY, Weiner JP, et al. Clinical outcomes after bariatric surgery: a five-year matched cohort analysis in seven US states. Obes Surg 2012;22(5):749–63.

22. Sugerman HJ, Wolfe LG, Sica DA, et al. Diabetes and hypertension in severe obesity and effects of gastric bypass-induced weight loss. Ann Surg 2003;237(6):751–8.

23. Clark JM. The epidemiology of nonalcoholic fatty liver disease in adults. J Clin Gastroenterol 2006;40:S5–10.

24. Sanyal AJ. NASH: a global health problem. Hepatol Res 2011;41(7):670–4.

25. Stephen S, Baranova A, Younossi ZM. Nonalcoholic fatty liver disease and bariatric surgery. Expert Rev Gastroenterol Hepatol 2012;6(2):163–71.

26. Targher G, Arcaro G. Non-alcoholic fatty liver disease and increased risk of cardiovascular disease. Atherosclerosis 2007;191(2):235–40.

27. Targher G, Byrne CD, Lonardo A, et al. Nonalcoholic fatty liver disease and risk of incident cardiovascular disease: a meta-analysis of observational studies. J Hepatol 2016;65(3):589–600.

28. Adams LA, Lymp JF, Sauver JS, et al. The natural history of nonalcoholic fatty liver disease: a population-based cohort study. Gastroenterology 2005;129(1):113–21.

29. Rabl C, Campos GM. The impact of bariatric surgery on nonalcoholic steatohepatitis. Semin Liver Dis 2012;32(1):80–91.

30. Brolin RE, Bradley LJ, Taliwal RV. Unsuspected cirrhosis discovered during elective obesity operations. Arch Surg 1998;133(1):84–8.

31. Jan A, Narwaria M, Mahawar KK. A systematic review of bariatric surgery in patients with liver cirrhosis. Obes Surg 2015;25(8):1518–26.

What Bariatric Surgery Can Teach Us About Endoluminal Treatment of Obesity and Metabolic Disorders

Lee M. Kaplan, MD, PhD

KEYWORDS

- Bariatric surgery • Weight regulation • Diabetes mellitus • Medical devices
- Obesity • Metabolic function • Gut microbiota • Bile acids

KEY POINTS

- Bariatric surgery causes durable weight loss by altering the physiologic regulation of body fat mass, demonstrating the critical role of the gastrointestinal (GI) tract in regulating energy balance and metabolic function.
- Mechanical restriction and macronutrient malabsorption do not appreciably contribute to the effectiveness of bariatric surgery.
- Bariatric surgery provides long-term benefit for patients with diabetes, fatty liver disease, and other metabolic disorders, through both weight loss–dependent and –independent mechanisms.
- Development of less invasive means of mimicking the effects of bariatric surgery could provide substantial benefit for a much greater number of patients.
- The mechanisms of action of bariatric surgery provides a valuable roadmap for the successful development and use of endoscopic, surgicomimetic therapies for obesity and related metabolic disorders.

INTRODUCTION

Of all the currently available treatments for obesity, bariatric surgery has by far the greatest efficacy. For the most commonly used procedures, vertical sleeve gastrectomy (VSG) and Roux-en-Y gastric bypass (RYGB), initial average weight loss is in the range of 35%, with approximately 75% to 80% of this weight loss maintained over an extended period, yielding an average weight loss in the range of 25% at

Disclosure: The author serves as a scientific consultant to Ethicon, Fractyl, Gelesis, GI Dynamics, Janssen, Kaleido, MedImmune, Medtronic, Merck, Novo Nordisk, Rhythm, USGI Medical, and Zafgen.
Obesity, Metabolism and Nutrition Institute, Massachusetts General Hospital, 149 13th Street, Room 8219, Boston, MA 02129, USA
E-mail address: LMKaplan@mgh.harvard.edu

10 years.[1] In addition, these gastrointestinal (GI) procedures have profound effects on metabolic disorders more broadly, inducing full or partial remission of diabetes and improvements in obstructive sleep apnea, fatty liver disease, hypertension, and dyslipidemia that are well beyond what is typically achieved with other antiobesity treatments.[2,3] In typical patients with severe obesity and 1 or more comorbidities, bariatric surgery is associated with a dramatic decrease in overall mortality and mortality from diabetes, cardiovascular disease, and cancer.[4] Despite these profound benefits, use of these procedures is severely limited. In the United States, approximately 200,000 patients undergo bariatric procedures each year, representing approximately 0.25% of all adults with obesity. This limited use reflects the invasive nature of bariatric surgery, potential complications, high cost, and incomplete reimbursement. These concerns are amplified by 2 additional factors: misunderstanding of both the pathophysiologic basis of obesity and the ability of surgery to ameliorate that pathophysiology. Surgery is widely perceived as forcing people to lose weight by limiting the amount of food that they can eat or the intestine's ability to absorb ingested nutrients. If these were the mechanisms, the outcomes would be very poor, with insatiable hunger and unrelenting cravings the price of a healthier weight. This article shows that these are not the mechanisms, and perpetual misery is not the cost. Instead, bariatric surgery induces global changes in the powerful and complex network of mechanisms that determine and defend the body's energy stores: the overall mass of body fat that is our living fuel tank. Obesity results from a combination of powerful environmental forces that induce the body to store an excess amount of fat, directly causing, exacerbating, and/or increasing the risk of developing more than 200 complicating or comorbid, diseases. Changes associated with modernization of the human environment have dramatically increased the number and intensity of these obesogenic forces over the past 150 years. Although genetics determine people's susceptibility to these forces, few people are genetically resistant to obesity, and that resistance often fades with the normal effects of maturity, childbirth, and aging.

During the past 2 decades, much has been learned about the physiologic mechanisms and neurohumoral circuits underlying the normal and abnormal control of body fat mass, and the genes and mechanisms that determine susceptibility to obesity.[5] However, the specific mechanisms by which changes in the modern environment induce and maintain obesity in susceptible individuals remain largely unknown. Nonetheless, the unique efficacy and durability of bariatric operations provides a positive control, a roadmap that could lead to a better understanding of the pathophysiology of obesity and guide the development of new, more effective strategies for its prevention and treatment. At a minimum, the profound effects of surgery, and the more recent recognition that these effects are grounded in physiology rather than physics, demonstrate the critical role of the GI tract in regulating and maintaining appropriate homeostasis in energy balance, fat mass, and metabolic function. Until the cellular and molecular mechanisms of these effects are more fully understood, finding less invasive means of manipulating the GI tract to induce the physiologic effects of surgery will likely provide the greatest near-term opportunity for such surgicomimetic treatment. Many early attempts at developing effective endoscopic treatments have failed. In some cases, these failures have resulted from unanticipated adverse events, but, in most cases, minimally invasive devices and procedures have not reproduced the dramatic benefits of surgery. Misunderstanding of the mechanisms by which bariatric surgery works can take clinicians down the wrong development path as they attempt to copy the physics without adequate attention to the physiology. Failure to recognize the multiplicity of manipulations and mechanisms inherent in most common bariatric procedures may blind clinicians to the need for combinations of less invasive treatments to achieve the power of surgery. Less invasive therapies do not need to be equal to surgery to provide important clinical value, but better understanding of how surgery works will almost certainly facilitate the path to devices and procedures that mimic the important benefits of surgery with profiles that allow for cost-effective treatment of a much larger portion of people with obesity, diabetes, and other metabolic disorders.

This review article summarizes current understanding of body weight and metabolic regulation and its implications for the causes and potential solutions to obesity and related diseases. It describes what is known about how surgery influences these metabolic processes and highlights specific cellular and molecular mechanisms induced by bariatric surgery that have recently been uncovered. In addition, recognizing that the effectiveness of surgery underscores the important metabolic regulatory role of the GI tract generally, it discusses how better understanding of surgical mechanisms could guide the development of new, more effective, and scalable GI-targeted therapies for these epidemic metabolic disorders, with particular attention to the development of effective endoscopic approaches.

REGULATION OF ENERGY BALANCE

There are 2 competing models of the regulation of human energy balance, fat mass, and body weight. The first and most widely held model is based on the voluntary regulation of calorie intake and expenditure, with obesity resulting primarily from a combination of overeating and inadequate energy expenditure from physical activity.[6] According to this model, the human body uses all absorbed calories, either to perform cellular or physical work (including cellular growth and regeneration) or to store as body fat. This model predicts that there is little internal, or autonomic, regulation of energy balance and little opportunity to dump excess calories other than by means of physical exercise.

The second model of energy regulation is based on regulation of energy balance as a homeostatic control system, with the body seeking to maintain some form of appropriate balance in the setting of varied environmental conditions and influences.[7] Under this model, ingestive behaviors and energy expenditure are regulated in response to physiologic state and metabolic demands. Modest, or even immodest, changes in food intake or physical activity are sensed by the endogenous regulatory machinery and compensatory mechanisms activated to maintain energy homeostasis. Under conditions of perceived energy deficit, this regulatory system induces increased food intake by increasing hunger, enhancing the reward value of nutrient-rich, high-calorie foods, and decreasing satiation and satiety. Nonessential energy expenditure is reduced, leading to a positive energy balance, net energy storage, and increased volume and mass of white adipose tissue, which is the body's organ of energy storage. In contrast, under conditions of perceived energy sufficiency or excess, the reverse occurs, with decreased hunger, decreased reward value of food, enhanced satiation and satiety, and increased energy expenditure. This facultative increase in energy expenditure occurs through enhanced thermogenesis (oxidation of circulating and stored fats, generating heat that is radiated into the environment) and increased involuntary physical activity (nonexercise activity thermogenesis, including fidgeting).

These divergent models have important implications for the prevention and treatment of obesity. Under the first, calorie-centric, model, obesity is predicted to result directly from excess caloric ingestion or inadequate physical activity. Its proponents suggest that, in modern society, increased food availability leads to an increase in ingested calories, and the decreased necessity for physical activity leads to decreased caloric expenditure, together generating a positive energy imbalance, increased fat mass, and weight gain. Thus, under this model, the proposed solution is to eat fewer calories and increase physical activity. Because both of these behaviors are perceived to be fully under voluntary control, the high and growing prevalence of obesity suggests an epidemic failure of personal responsibility, generating the perception that people with obesity are intellectually, morally, or psychologically compromised and reinforcing the prevalent stigma against such individuals.

Under the second model, the body aims to maintain energy stores (ie, white adipose tissue mass) appropriate to the body's physiologic state and uses regulation of both behavior and metabolic activity to do so. Obesity results from influences (endogenous or environmental) that cause this autonomic regulatory system to seek and defend inappropriately increased energy stores, thereby increasing fat mass and body weight and size. This model predicts that the most effective treatment of obesity will result from changing metabolic physiology so that the body's desired energy stores are reduced to a more normal, physiologically appropriate range. Effective prevention strategies would be designed to block the influences that alter metabolic physiology in the first place.

Although both models likely contribute to the overall control of energy balance and the current epidemic of obesity, there is increasing evidence of the dominance of the second, autonomic regulatory model. As described later, some of the strongest evidence results from the profound beneficial effects of bariatric procedures and the growing understanding of their mechanisms of action. These mechanisms demonstrate the prominent role of the GI tract in the normal regulation of energy balance and metabolic function. They show the value of GI-targeted interventions in the effective prevention and treatment of obesity and related metabolic disorders. In addition, they can provide critical guidance to gastroenterologists and to those who seek to develop endoscopic, radiologic, pharmacologic, or dietary therapies that mimic the mechanisms and effectiveness of bariatric surgery.

WHAT CAUSES OBESITY?

Obesity, like virtually all diseases, is caused by environmental influences acting on biologically susceptible individuals. Numerous studies have shown that predisposition or resistance to obesity is largely determined by genetic background.[8] There are at least 10 genes in which mutations lead directly to obesity, but these monogenic obesities are exceeding rare.[9] Far more commonly, modest variations in or around more than 100 other genes have been shown to alter an individual's predisposition to obesity, and those whose genome includes multiple obesity-predisposing polymorphisms are likely to be at substantially increased risk.[8] However, as has been widely noted, the rapid increase in the prevalence and severity of obesity cannot be explained by recent changes in people's genetic background, so other factors must be operative. The obvious and most likely cause is a profound change in the modern environment, but what are these environmental factors? According to the widely held calorie imbalance model of fat mass regulation, obesity is caused by the combination of increased availability and therefore consumption of calories, combined with reduced physical activity–mediated energy expenditure. Proponents of this model suggest that evolution has favored protection against starvation rather than protection against obesity, with food scarcity serving as the major barrier to obesity in earlier times. However, this model has several flaws. During earlier times, when the human population was substantially smaller and natural plant-based and animal-based foods almost certainly as plentiful as they are now, scarcity-based barriers to excessive food intake would likely have provided inadequate protection. Although more physical labor was likely required to obtain nutrients, recent studies of primitive hunter-gatherer tribes show that the greater activity-based energy expenditure is offset by decreased thermogenesis, such that the daily total energy expenditure (TEE) of these naturally thin hunter-gatherers is no greater than that of sedentary members of modern society. Many studies have shown that even very modest selective advantage is sufficient for allelic exclusion over several generations, and the adverse physiologic effects of excessive body fat is certainly a sufficient selective disadvantage.[10,11]

It is more likely that changes in the modern environment affect the normal physiologic apparatus that regulates energy balance and determines body fat stores. Such influences need not be calorie dependent; they only need to influence the signaling and biochemical mechanisms that underlie normal regulation of fat mass. Although researchers have not defined all of the potential environmental contributors, changes in 6 domains that are common to modernization in nearly all societies likely contribute to the ubiquitous growth of obesity across the globe:

- Alterations of the chemical content of foods, including processing to remove natural ingredients, add new chemical ingredients, decrease fiber and plant-based oligosaccharides, and increased nutrient homogeneity
- Increased availability and use of labor-saving machinery, which can lead to muscle dysfunction and diminished muscle-derived regulators of energy balance
- Sleep deprivation
- Disruption of circadian rhythms
- Increased speed and stress of modern life
- Obesity-promoting medications, including many used to treat common metabolic, cardiovascular, autoimmune, psychiatric, and infectious diseases

BARIATRIC SURGICAL PROCEDURES

There are multiple effective types of bariatric and metabolic surgery, each with different anatomic and clinical implications. In addition, within each primary type of surgery, there are multiple versions that differ in subtle and not so subtle ways. This article focuses primarily on the major types, because they have generated the most clinical experience and have generally been subjected to the most carefully executed and controlled studies. All of these operations are now routinely performed using a laparoscopic approach, which has been shown to reduce hospital stay, the duration of bed rest, and the risk of wound infections and abdominal wall hernias.[12] Otherwise, clinical outcomes after laparoscopically performed operations seem to be the same as for procedures performed via (open) laparotomy.

Roux-en-Y Gastric Bypass

This operation, depicted in **Fig. 1**A, includes separation of a portion of the gastric cardia from the remainder of the stomach to create a small (typically 30–50 mL volume) gastric pouch, and transection of the proximal jejunum to midjejunum. The distal small bowel is brought up and anastomosed to the gastric pouch, providing an exit from the pouch directly into the midjejunum. The proximal side of the transected jejunum is anastomosed to the jejunum further down, providing an exit pathway for this biliopancreatic (BP) limb, which contains pancreatic and biliary secretions into the duodenum, as well as secretions and sloughed mucosa from the now nutrient-bare distal stomach (gastric remnant), duodenum, and proximal jejunum. As a result, after RYGB, ingested nutrients pass from the mouth (interacting with the oral mucosa and taste buds and activating the cephalic phase of the response to ingestion) to the

A	B	C	D	E
Roux-en-Y Gastric Bypass	Biliopancreatic Diversion	Duodenal Switch	Vertical Sleeve Gastrectomy	Adjustable Gastric Banding

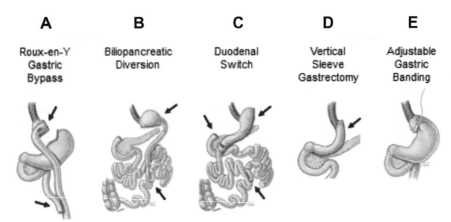

Fig. 1. The anatomy of bariatric surgery. (*A*) Roux-en-Y gastric bypass. (*B*) Biliopancreatic diversion. (*C*) Duodenal switch version of biliopancreatic diversion. (*D*) Vertical sleeve gastrectomy. (*E*) Adjustable gastric band. The arrows indicate critical anatomic changes or device implantations characteristic of each procedure. (*Reprinted with* permission, Cleveland Clinic Center for Medical Art & Photography © 2006-2016. All Rights Reserved.)

esophagus to the small gastric pouch. They are then rapidly passed directly to the midjejunal Roux (or alimentary) limb for digestion, absorption, and further processing. The contents of the BP limb mix with those of the alimentary limb at the jejunojejunal (J-J) anastomosis, passing together into the common channel for further digestion, absorption/reabsorption, or passage to the colon for ultimate excretion. Even though it is now performed less commonly than VSG (discussed later), RYGB is considered the gold standard bariatric procedure, with an excellent risk-benefit profile for the treatment of obesity, type 2 diabetes, and several other obesity-related metabolic disorders.[2,3,13]

Biliopancreatic Diversion

Conceptually, the BP diversion (BPD; see **Fig. 1**B) is similar to that of an RYGB, with creation of a diminished gastric pouch that empties directly into the distal small intestine and a BP limb that joins the alimentary limb more distally. In the case of the standard BPD, the gastric antrum and pylorus are resected, leaving a much larger gastric pouch than is created during an RYGB but no gastric remnant at the proximal end of the BP limb. Both the alimentary and BP limbs are substantially longer than after an RYGB, leaving a relative short (typically 75–100 cm) common channel between the J-J anastomosis and the ileocecal valve. A variant of the BPD, commonly termed the duodenal switch (DS) procedure (see **Fig. 1**C), includes creation of a narrow tube-like stomach by resection of the greater curvature of the stomach, and preservation of the pylorus between the stomach and alimentary limb. The small intestinal anatomy of the DS is essentially the same as in the standard version of the BPD. Because of the particularly long duodenal-jejunal bypass segment and short common channel, BPD is associated with an increased risk of malabsorption of macronutrients, as well as micronutrients (eg, minerals, vitamins, and other organic compounds) and therapeutic medications that depend on metabolism, transport, and/or absorption in the proximal small intestine. Because of the large interindividual variation in small intestinal length and function, the lengths of alimentary and BP limbs and common channel that provide optimal benefit with minimal malabsorptive risk are not well defined. Malabsorptive adverse effects can often be prevented or ameliorated by creating a longer (eg, $\geq$100 cm) common channel. However, because of the greater risk of associated metabolic and malabsorptive complications, BPD accounts for only about 2% of bariatric procedures.

Vertical Sleeve Gastrectomy

With its greater efficacy than RYGB, BPD, and its DS variant have been preferentially used by some surgeons for the treatment of patients with severe obesity (eg, patients with BMI >60 kg/m^2). However, because of the risks of major surgery in many of these heavier patients, several surgeons have opted for a 2-stage DS procedure, with the easier, and apparently safer, resection of the stomach vertical sleeve gastrectomy (VSG) allowing for initial weight loss, followed after several months by creation of the intestinal bypass anatomy. The dramatic effect observed in the first-phase operation (VSG) led several surgeons to propose using the VSG as an isolated bariatric procedure (see **Fig. 1**C). This operation involves resection of the full greater curve of the stomach, leaving behind a banana-shaped or tube-shaped stomach. Despite loss of the grinding, or mill, function of the stomach and maintaining the pylorus intact, patients who have undergone a VSG show substantially more rapid gastric emptying. Because of its relative ease and excellent efficacy, the VSG has become the most commonly performed bariatric procedure, accounting for approximately 50% of all such operations worldwide and at least 65% of those performed in the United States.

Adjustable Gastric Banding

Adjustable gastric banding (AGB) (see **Fig. 1**E) is the latest in a series of bariatric procedures designed to limit the effective size of the stomach, including horizontal, vertical, and vertical-banded gastroplasties. Using one of 2 FDA-approved adjustable banding devices, an AGB procedure includes placement of, the flexible, hollow device around the gastric cardia. The band is linked through an imbedded filling tube to a port placed subcutaneously in the abdominal wall. Filling of the device narrows the passage through which ingested food passes from the distal esophagus/gastric cardia into the gastric body, slowing the passage and potentially increasing ingestion-associated luminal pressure and/or wall stretch and tension proximal to the device, thereby stimulating mural mechanoreceptors. Initially very popular because of its easy placement and excellent initial safety profile, AGB has lost favor in recent years because of the modest associated weight loss, absence of weight loss–independent metabolic benefit, and risk of erosion into or through the gastric wall. At present, AGB accounts for approximately 5% of bariatric procedures in the United States and worldwide.

MECHANISMS OF WEIGHT LOSS AFTER BARIATRIC SURGERY

Beginning in the 1950s, several surgeons began to explore means of manipulating the GI tract to induce weight loss. Based on the then-prevalent understanding of energy balance and obesity, they hypothesized that limiting food ingestion, or preventing absorption of ingested calorie-containing macronutrients, would lead to negative energy balance and weight loss. The first commonly used procedure, the jejunoileal bypass (JIB), was designed to induce macronutrient malabsorption.[14] That it proved a highly effective means of inducing long-term weight loss reinforced the notion that reduction of net calorie intake (calories ingested minus calories excreted in the stool) was its dominant mechanism of action. In the 1960s, 1970s, and 1980s, many additional operations were designed and tested, some based on limiting the size of the stomach to restrict allowable food intake (eg, various forms of gastroplasty), and some, such as RYGB and BPD, combining such so-called "restrictive" and "malabsorptive" characteristics.[15] That some of these operations caused macronutrient (calorie) malabsorption is unquestioned. However, even the earliest studies of JIB in human patients and animal models showed a postoperative reduction in food intake.[16,17] This observation stood in contrast with the situation with disease-induced or surgery-induced short bowel syndrome, in which malabsorption is associated with a dramatic increase in appetitive drive and food intake as the body attempts to counteract the obligate loss of calories in the stool. That this does not occur in calorie-wasting bariatric procedures was the first clue that they work through other mechanisms. Now 60 years later, it can be concluded that the dominant mechanisms of action of these procedures depend on their ability to ameliorate the physiologic dysregulation of energy balance and fat mass that causes obesity in the first place.

What is the evidence? As noted, patients who undergo bariatric surgery typically experience profound decreases in hunger and hedonic drives to eating, along with enhanced postprandial satiety.[18] These responses are opposite to what would be expected with restriction or malabsorption, which typically lead to increased hunger, craving, and decreased satiety.[18] These differences in the effects of calorie restriction and bariatric surgery on appetitive drives are also reflected in differences in levels of appetite-regulating peptides. After calorie restriction or conditions of severe malabsorption, circulating levels of ghrelin, an appetite-promoting hormone, are increased, and circulating levels of several appetite-suppressing hormones, including glucagon-like peptide 1 (GLP-1), peptide tyrosine-tyrosine (PYY), amylin, and cholecystokinin (CCK), are decreased.[19,20] After VSG, RYGB, BPD, and many other forms of bariatric surgery, the levels of these peptide hormones all change in the opposite direction.[21] These observations strongly suggest that, under conditions of calorie restriction or malabsorption, the body attempts to defend the original energy stores, activating mechanisms that counter the effect of the initial weight loss. In contrast, immediately after bariatric surgery (before significant weight loss), the body behaves in a manner that drives weight loss, as though it is seeking a lower fat mass target. Recent studies of bariatric surgery in rodent models confirm this interpretation. In these studies, diet-induced obese rats or mice underwent VSG or RYGB. After surgery-induced weight loss and stabilization at the lower weight, the animals were then calorie restricted to induce further weight loss. When they were subsequently allowed to eat ad libitum, they overate and regained the weight lost from the dietary restriction, returning to their original postoperative weights.[22] These studies show that, even after bariatric surgery, these animals are not physically prevented from eating more; they choose to eat less as they seek a lower fat mass, but, if challenged by further dietary restriction, they overeat to defend that new, lower postoperative fat mass target. Although these studies have not been reproduced in human patients (and are not likely to be tried in the near future), there is other evidence that surgery works by altering physiology rather than ingestive or absorptive capacity. Women who become pregnant after bariatric surgery increase food consumption and gain weight appropriately.[23,24] Thus, they have the capacity to eat and absorb more but, in the absence of pregnancy, their bodies choose not to. Together, these observations show that bariatric surgery alters the regulation of body energy stores (fat mass) in a manner that promotes a lower target fat mass. However, as powerful as bariatric surgery is, its effects can be overcome by the fat mass regulatory impact of pregnancy and lactation.

ANATOMIC DETERMINANTS OF RESPONSE

One of the great challenges in understanding the mechanisms of action of bariatric and metabolic surgery is the apparently similar responses to disparate anatomic manipulations. VSG, RYGB, and BPD generate similar effects on adiposity and type 2 diabetes, suggesting that different parts of the GI tract can contribute to its regulation of metabolic function. Considering first the RYGB, this operation can be considered to include 6 major effects of the altered postoperative anatomy:

1. Decreased size of the gastric reservoir, with potential changes (augmentation) of the activation of mechanoreceptors in response to food intake.
2. Partial gastric vagotomy necessitated by transection of the proximal stomach containing vagal nerve ramifications in the creation of the gastric pouch.
3. Diversion of the ingested nutrient stream away from the distal gastric remnant, where it can no longer interact with the bulk of the oxyntic (endocrine) mucosa of the stomach.
4. Diversion of the ingested nutrient stream away from the duodenum and proximal jejunum, where it can no longer mix or interact with pancreaticobiliary secretions, the microbiota, or the mucosa of the proximal small bowel. Mixture of the contents of the 2 limbs occurs more distally, allowing these interactions to occur in the distal jejunum and ileum.
5. Exposure of the proximal small intestine to GI and BP secretions unaltered by and unbound to ingested nutrients and their metabolic products.
6. Exposure of the mid and distal small intestine to less completely digested nutrients.

Which of these anatomic changes, alone or in combination, are responsible for the diverse biological effects of RYGB remains controversial. There is substantial evidence that physiologic changes in signaling from the duodenum as a result of the nutrient diversion (4 and 5 in the list) contribute to the beneficial effects of RYGB on obesity and type 2 diabetes, leading to what has been termed the foregut model of bariatric surgical action. There is also evidence supporting the importance of altered ileal L cell–mediated signaling (6 in the list), leading to the so-called hindgut model of action. Further consideration of these models and their application to the effects of surgery on energy balance, fat mass, carbohydrate and lipid metabolism, and their associated diseases is described later.

EFFECT OF SURGERY ON METABOLIC DISEASES

In their review of bariatric surgery outcomes, Hanipah and Schauer describe the powerful beneficial effects of bariatric surgery on type 2 diabetes, sleep apnea, nonalcoholic fatty liver disease, and other metabolic complications of obesity (See Zubaidah Nor Hanipah and Philip R. Schauer, "Surgical Treatment of Obesity and Diabetes," in this issue). The effects of VSG, RYGB, and BPD on type 2 diabetes provide a particularly important window on the role of the GI tract in the regulation of metabolic function. As early as 1955, surgeons recognized that type 2 diabetes rapidly improved after jejunoileal bypass, and in 1995, Pories and colleagues[25] showed almost complete remission of diabetes in a cohort of patients undergoing RYGB. These observations, which have been confirmed in several randomized controlled studies, have recently led to the incorporation of bariatric surgery into the standard guidelines for treating type 2 diabetes.[26]

However, despite these clinical advances, the precise mechanisms by which bariatric surgery alters carbohydrate and lipid metabolism remain poorly understood. Several studies have shown that the enhanced postoperative secretion of GLP-1 enhances pancreatic insulin secretion, consistent with the known effect of this incretin hormone. Surgery improves insulin sensitivity as well, but the degree to which this improvement is independent of postoperative weight loss remains unclear.

The effects of AGB on type 2 diabetes are directly correlated with, and apparently dependent on, weight loss after this procedure.[27] However, the improvement in diabetes after VSG, RYGB, and BPD appears to include both weight loss–dependent and weight loss–independent mechanisms. Despite the impressive early postoperative remission, several recent studies have shown that this rapid improvement can be accounted for by the dramatic reduction in food intake in the several weeks after these operations. Very-low-calorie diets and diets matched to those prescribed after bariatric surgery exert similar effects on blood glucose, insulin secretion, and insulin sensitivity.[28,29] In contrast, studies in rodent models have shown that the long-term benefits of RYGB on glucose homeostasis are substantially greater than those induced by the same amount of weight loss from dietary restriction alone.[30] The mechanisms of this weight loss–independent and food intake–independent improvement in type 2 diabetes should help elucidate the normal metabolic regulatory role of the gut. However, at present, even the primary site of this regulatory activity within the intestine is controversial. Human and rodent studies of RYGB and BPD suggest an important role of bypassing the duodenum, and cannulation and refeeding of the normally bypassed BP limb after RYGB has been shown to reverse many of the effects of this operation.[31] However, these operations are complex and include manipulation of the stomach and (with BPD) distal small intestine. An important role of the duodenum is supported by studies of the effects of isolated duodenal manipulation using duodenojejunal bypass (DJB) in rats, endoluminal duodenal liner implantation in humans and rats, and duodenal mucosal ablation in humans and rats.[32–35] However, the duodenum need not be the only relevant segment of the bowel for regulation of glucose homeostasis.

VSG, which does not change the path of nutrient flow or bypass the duodenum, induces most of the same metabolic effects as RYGB, suggesting other segments of the gut are involved. Many investigators have postulated that, by bypassing a portion of the small intestine, more undigested nutrients reach the distal ileum, which contains the highest concentration of GLP-1–secreting L cells within the small intestine (there are even higher concentrations in the colon). Perhaps the accelerated transit of ingested nutrients through the stomach after VSG has a similar effect, but this is highly speculative. Small intestinal resection studies have shown substantial excess digestive and absorptive capacity of this organ, and it is not clear that undigested nutrients reach the ileum in greater concentration after VSG or RYGB. It is known that circulating GLP-1 levels are substantially increased after all of these procedures except AGB, but, as noted earlier, the primary anatomic source of this increased secretion has not been established. The patterns of bile acid transport and reuptake in the distal ileum, the stimulatory effects of bile acids on L-cell GLP-1 secretion, and the beneficial effects of bile diversion and direct bile acid instillation into the distal small bowel all support a role for the ileum in the metabolic improvements after bariatric surgery, but proof of its role is still elusive.

Considering all of the available data, it seems that multiple segments of the gut may contribute to the GI regulation of energy balance and lipid and carbohydrate metabolism, perhaps with built-in redundancies that account for the similar benefits of multiple anatomically distinct interventions. Based on the anatomic and functional changes induced by bariatric surgery, and the several likely cellular and molecular mediators thus far identified, it makes most sense to consider the gut regulation of metabolic function from the lumen outward. Whether by alteration in pathways of flow, speed of gastric emptying, mucosal removal or mucosal inaccessibility, each type of bariatric surgery seems to alter the profile of nutrients and their digestive products, secreted enzymes, pH, bile acids, and microbiota and their metabolic products at every level of the gut from the stomach to the colon. Within each gut segment, the interaction of these altered contents with receptors and other sensors on or within the intestinal mucosa, which itself may be altered by the surgery, leads to widespread changes in humoral, neural, and immune cell–mediated signals emanating from the gut (**Fig. 2**).

PHYSIOLOGIC MECHANISMS OF SURGICAL ACTION
Appetitive Drives and Appetite-Regulating Hormones

As noted earlier, VSG, RYGB, and BPD all lead to diminished appetite, by decreasing hunger and the hedonic effects or reward value of food, and increasing intrameal satiation and postprandial satiety.[36–38] In addition, in both human patients and animal models, these operations induce profound changes in food preference, with increased predilection for and consumption of foods lower in sugar and fat content and lower in calorie density.[39] These effects are likely mediated, at least in part, by altered neurohumoral signaling after bariatric surgery. Circulating postprandial levels of the satiety-inducing enteroendocrine cell–secreted hormones GLP-1 and PYY increase

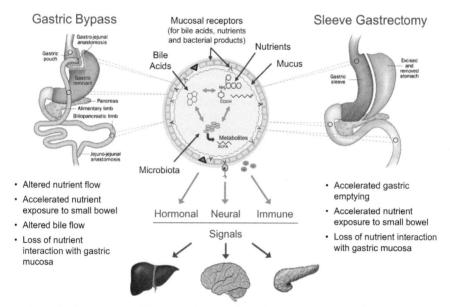

Fig. 2. Bariatric surgery and the gastrointestinal regulation of metabolic function. In every segment of the gastrointestinal tract, luminal contents interact with receptors and other signaling molecules expressed in mucosal epithelial cells or neighboring cells. These interactions generate or alter molecular signals that emanate from the gut. These gut-derived signals then communicate with the brain and with metabolically active peripheral tissues, including the liver, muscle, and brown and white fat themselves. After sleeve gastrectomy, gastric bypass and other bariatric operations, the molecular composition of luminal contents is altered at every level of the gut from the stomach to rectum. These changes alter the interactions with mucosal receptors and other sensors, leading to changes in the signals emanating from the gut that regulate body fat, energy balance and intermediary metabolism. The similar effects of VSG and RYGB suggest that no one anatomic manipulation is uniquely required for the observed benefits of these operations. While removal of gastric or intestinal mucosa, bypassing the duodenum, accelerating nutrient emptying in to the small bowel, or creating a shorter pathway through the small intestine into the ileum and colon may contribute to the physiological effects of these procedures, no single manipulation may be either necessary or sufficient for the key metabolic benefits of these operations.

substantially after each of these operations, and circulating levels of satiety-inducing peptides CCK and amylin have been shown to increase after several of them.[40] In addition, circulating levels of ghrelin, a strong appetite-stimulating hormone secreted by gastric endocrine cells, are frequently suppressed after these procedures.[41]

Despite these important observations about the effects of surgery on these gut-derived appetite-regulating hormones, this cannot be the whole, or even the primary, mechanism of surgical action. First, it is not yet clear what promotes increased secretion of the appetite-suppressing hormones. For example, how does surgery cause intestinal L cells to increase their secretion of GLP-1 and PYY? There is some suggestion that bile acids may play a role, but these data are far from conclusive.[42] Even less is known about the means by which surgery affects intestinal CCK secretion or pancreatic beta cell secretion of amylin. It is not yet known which of the relevant enteroendocrine cells are responsible for the enhanced secretion. L cells are present (in different concentrations) throughout the small intestine and colon but their phenotypic and physiologic characteristics differ.

Although concentrations of these satiety-inducing peptides increase dramatically after surgery, and circulating ghrelin levels are blunted, it is not clear to what degree these changes account for the weight loss and improved metabolic function. Deletion of the genes encoding the GLP-1 receptor or ghrelin has no appreciable effect on outcomes after VSG or RYGB, suggesting that these peptides are not required for the effects of these operations.[43–45] Nonetheless, given the complex regulation of energy balance and metabolic function, these observations do not exclude an important role for these peptides under normal circumstances, only that their function can be complemented by other mechanisms when they are absent.

Energy Expenditure

As noted earlier, calorie restriction–induced weight loss is associated with decreased TEE, presumably as part of a compensatory mechanism to limit weight loss and defend the target fat mass.[46] In contrast, RYGB and BPD are associated with increased TEE, which contributes to the weight loss.[47,48] This response is particularly important in rodent models in which the increased energy expenditure accounts for between 50% and 90% of the observed weight loss after these operations.[30] The enhanced energy expenditure does not seem to be from increased physical activity. It results from increased diet-induced thermogenesis, derived at least in part from enhanced activation of brown and/or beige fat. In human patients, this effect is more modest, accounting for less than 10% of the total weight loss. Nonetheless, the ability of these operations to increase stimulatory signals to thermogenic tissues and to blunt or reverse the energy conservation associated with diet-induced weight loss seems to be an important component of their mechanism. In contrast with the diversionary (bypass) procedures, VSG does not seem to induce an absolute increase in TEE; nonetheless, in rodent models, it clearly blunts the decreased energy expenditure seen after calorie restriction.[22] As with changes in appetite, the molecular mechanisms underlying the postoperative changes in energy expenditure remain poorly understood. Observed changes in circulating bile acid levels could play a role, as could changes in the gut microbiota (discussed later), but these mechanisms are more speculative than proven at present.

Regulation of Circadian Rhythms

Disruption of sleep and normal circadian rhythms disrupts normal metabolic regulation, leading to obesity and type 2 diabetes.[49–52] In rodent models, RYGB and VSG have been shown to influence circadian regulation in a manner that may contribute to their beneficial metabolic effects. The extent to which these circadian effects contribute to the overall metabolic benefits of these operations remains unclear. Moreover, the relationship between bariatric surgery and circadian regulation seems complex. One study has shown that weight loss after RYGB is blunted among third-shift workers, suggesting that disruption of circadian rhythms seems to partially interfere with the metabolic effects of surgery.[53]

Bile Acids

Several independent lines of evidence implicate bile acids as important mediators of the metabolic benefits of bariatric surgery. These signaling lipids, through activation of the cell surface bile acid receptor TGR5, stimulate GLP-1 secretion from intestinal L cells and enhance thermogenesis in brown and beige adipocytes.[42,54] RYGB, VSG, and BPD all induce increased concentrations of bile acids circulating in the peripheral blood, where they have access to these cell surface receptors.[55–57] Farsenoid X receptor (FXR), the predominant nuclear bile acid receptor, has also been shown to play a role in the response to bariatric surgery, because mice whose FXR gene is deleted are unable to maintain weight loss after VSG.[58] Isolated biliary diversion, a surgical procedure that shunts bile from the gallbladder or bile duct directly into the distal jejunum, induces many of the same effects as more classic bariatric procedures.[59] In both human patients and rodent models, biliary diversion induces substantial weight loss and improved glucose homeostasis. These effects can be seen, to a more limited extent, by direct instillation of taurinylated ursodeoxycholic acid, a bile acid present in high concentrations in the intestinal lumen and plasma, into the jejunum.[60] However, little is known about the roles of specific bile acids in the responses to bariatric surgery, or the manner in which these operations each alter the relative concentrations of different bile acids in different sites within the enterohepatic circulation and in the peripheral blood. With more than 100 different bile acids synthesized and maintained in the human body, each with unique biochemical, transport, receptor-binding, and activation characteristics, it is likely that different bile acid species play distinct roles in the regulation of metabolic function. Work to elucidate these differential effects is still in its infancy.

Microbiota

Within the past decade, the availability of new and more powerful sequencing and analytical tools has rapidly accelerated the ability to characterize the intestinal microbiota and helped elucidate its many contributions to host biology. Among its contributions, the microbiota seems to exert important effects on host metabolic function, strongly influencing the development and treatment of obesity, type 2 diabetes, and nonalcoholic fatty liver disease, among others.[61] Several recent studies have shown dramatic changes in the ecological structure and biological activities within the microbiota in response to RYGB and VSG, with enhancement in the prevalence of microbes associated with improved host metabolic function, such as *Akkermansia muciniphila* and *Roseburia* spp.[62] Two studies have shown that transfer of the microbiota from RYGB-treated mice or human subjects into unoperated, germ-free mice transmits a significant portion of the decreased adiposity associated with RYGB.[62,63] The decreased body weight in RYGB microbiota–recipient mice occurs despite increased food intake in these animals, with evidence suggesting that the RYGB microbiota contributes to the increased host energy expenditure observed after this operation. In addition, transfer of the RYGB microbiota induces changes in the distribution of short-chain fatty acids identical to that seen after RYGB in the donor mice. Transfer of microbiota from human RYGB patients to germ-free mice also leads to increased concentrations of circulating bile acids in the recipient animals, similar to the bile acid response in the operated donor mice and human patients. All of these changes are specific to the microbiota from RYGB-treated animals and patients, showing an important contribution of the microbiota to the metabolic responses to bariatric surgery. Nonetheless, whether the observed changes in short-chain fatty acids or bile acids are the primary molecular mechanisms by which the microbiota exert their metabolic effects is not yet known.

Integrated Responses to Bariatric Surgery

Although bariatric surgery induces widespread changes in metabolic function and activates multiple distinct mechanisms, the overall physiologic effects of these operations seem to reflect a global response that integrates these various individual changes. The postoperative changes in the intestinal lumen lead to altered signaling to the mucosa, which in turn seems to alter neurohumoral signaling from the gut to the brain, brown fat, liver, pancreas, and white fat, leading to the observed global changes in metabolic function. However, even within the lumen, the various contributing mechanisms seem to be interrelated. Although changes in nutrient metabolites, bile acids, microbiota, and their metabolic products can individually influence the host, it is also apparent that each influences the others. Changes in microbiota after bariatric surgery influence the concentration and distribution of bile acids, which in turn influence the microbial ecology. Similarly, there is a 2-way interaction between ingested nutrients and microbiota that regulates the metabolic products and signaling characteristics of both. There are interactions among nutrients, microbiota, and circadian rhythms that affect host metabolism. In addition, there are strong and complex bidirectional interactions between the intestinal lumen and (extraluminal) host that govern all aspects of both host and microbiota metabolism. In this context, trying to assign specific functions to individual molecules, cells, or intestinal segments seems less useful than identifying patterns, or signatures, of luminal and extraluminal signaling activity that correlate with important physiologic and clinical phenotypes or that predict therapeutic responses. These signatures could be valuable in discriminating the different mechanisms and outcomes of different bariatric procedures. They could serve as early markers of the efficacy and safety of novel GI-targeted metabolic therapies, their ability to mimic 1 or more aspects of bariatric surgery, or their likely effectiveness in individual patients.

IMPLICATIONS FOR ENDOSCOPIC TREATMENT OF OBESITY AND RELATED METABOLIC DISORDERS

The powerful therapeutic effects of bariatric surgery and the recognition of their physiologic basis has revealed the potential for effective, GI-targeted therapy for obesity, diabetes, fatty liver disease, and numerous other related metabolic disorders. Although the details of the underlying cellular and molecular mechanisms are not yet defined, and there is controversy about the relative contributions of different gut segments, what is already known has important implications for the development of novel therapies designed to exploit these mechanisms. For example, it is clear that the ratio of weight loss to improvement in glucose metabolism varies among different surgical procedures and endoscopic therapies. Some of these differences seem predictable, some less so. For weight loss, initial thoughts focused on the contributions of signals emanating from the duodenum and ileum. The success of the sleeve gastrectomy raises at least 2 new possibilities: (1) that the speed, or timing, of nutrient entry to the small intestinal lumen, or interaction with the intestinal mucosa, may have a strong influence on regulation of energy balance; and (2) that interactions within the stomach may be a major regulator of fat mass regulation. It is notable that, despite its powerful effect on type 2 diabetes, DJB is far less effective for the treatment of obesity.[32] The stomach is not manipulated by DJB, although bypassing the pylorus may still result in more rapid transit of ingested nutrients to the small intestine. Ileal interposition and duodenal mucosal ablation (resurfacing) have similar profiles, with far greater effects on glucose metabolism than energy balance.[33,64] The profile of the endoluminal duodenal liner is intermediate, but the placement of this device immediately distal to the pylorus, and the observation of substantially greater weight loss with a constrictor version of the device, suggest that some of the weight loss effects may result from placing an afterload that increases luminal pressure, wall tension, or stretch within the stomach.[34] Further support for an important role of the stomach in body weight regulation comes from recent studies of the Aspire Assist device, which seems to be particularly effective in inducing weight loss, and from early observations of the effects of left gastric embolization, which may provide a limited imitation of the mucosal loss inherent in VSG.[65,66] From the perspective of treating diabetes and perhaps other strictly metabolic disorders, these observations suggest that manipulation of the small bowel is key. However, it is necessary to better understand the large therapeutic benefit of VSG for diabetes, which although not as great as that of RYGB, is impressive nonetheless. Is this a metabolic effect of the loss of oxyntic (endocrine) mucosa in the greater curvature, or does it work through the small bowel by substantially increasing the speed of nutrient passage through the stomach?

However, amid all the ambiguity about mechanism, what is clear is that bariatric surgery works by altering the basic physiology regulating energy balance, energy storage, and defense of fat mass that underlies the development and effective treatment of obesity. It influences all inputs to energy balance, including hunger, food-seeking behaviors, hedonic drives, satiation and satiety, as well as regulation of energy expenditure in multiple tissues. Simultaneously, through common or independent mechanisms, it alters the regulation of metabolic signaling and intermediary metabolism that underlies the development and effective treatment of diabetes and related metabolic disorders. Surgery does not seem to work by restricting the amount of food ingested or the efficiency of absorption or energy harvest. In some operations, when malabsorption of micronutrients or macronutrients does occur, it should be considered an adverse effect, increasing the risk without providing substantial therapeutic benefit.

So what does this mean for development, testing, and clinical use of endoscopic therapies? Success is likely to come from reproducing the mechanisms underlying the therapeutic benefits of surgery. Obstruction, restriction, space-occupying devices, and intestinal resection seem unlikely to induce substantial long-term benefit unless they can be engineered to induce neurohumoral mechanisms that have thus far eluded the direct electrical stimulation, various forms of gastroplasty, and most endogastric devices tested.

The increasingly dire health, social, and economic consequences of obesity and its complications demand novel approaches to both prevention and therapy. Bariatric surgery shows the utility and power of GI-targeted therapies, and the public health benefits that could be provided by effective but less invasive GI manipulation are enormous. Understanding the means by which bariatric surgery generates its profound therapeutic benefits will facilitate the development of effective but less invasive means that achieve the same outcome. Misapprehension of those mechanisms is sure to lead down the wrong path, wasting valuable time, energy, and resources on approaches that ultimately fail to meet the needs of patients and society at large.

REFERENCES

1. Sjostrom L, Narbro K, Sjostrom CD, et al. Effects of bariatric surgery on mortality in Swedish obese subjects. N Engl J Med 2007;357(8):741–52.
2. Buchwald H, Avidor Y, Braunwald E, et al. Bariatric surgery: a systematic review and meta-analysis. JAMA 2004;292(14):1724–37.
3. Schauer PR, Kashyap SR, Wolski K, et al. Bariatric surgery versus intensive medical therapy in obese patients with diabetes. N Engl J Med 2012;366(17): 1567–76.
4. Arterburn DE, Olsen MK, Smith VA, et al. Association between bariatric surgery and long-term survival. JAMA 2015;313(1):62–70.
5. Berthoud HR, Morrison C. The brain, appetite, and obesity. Annu Rev Psychol 2008;59:55–92.
6. Davis C, Patte K, Levitan R, et al. From motivation to behaviour: a model of reward sensitivity, overeating, and food preferences in the risk profile for obesity. Appetite 2007;48(1):12–9.
7. Berthoud HR. Homeostatic and non-homeostatic pathways involved in the control of food intake and energy balance. Obesity 2006;14(Suppl 5):197S–200S.
8. Bradfield JP, Taal HR, Timpson NJ, et al. A genome-wide association meta-analysis identifies new childhood obesity loci. Nat Genet 2012;44(5):526–31.
9. Farooqi IS, O'Rahilly S. Monogenic obesity in humans. Annu Rev Med 2005;56: 443–58.
10. Pritchard JK, Cox NJ. The allelic architecture of human disease genes: common disease-common variant...or not? Hum Mol Genet 2002;11(20):2417–23.
11. Power ML, Schulkin J. Sex differences in fat storage, fat metabolism, and the health risks from obesity: possible evolutionary origins. Br J Nutr 2008;99(5): 931–40.
12. Schirmer B. Laparoscopic bariatric surgery. Surg Endosc 2006;20(Suppl 2): S450–5.
13. Neff KJ, le Roux CW. Bariatric surgery: a best practice article. J Clin Pathol 2013; 66(2):90–8.
14. Kremen AJ, Linner JH, Nelson CH. An experimental evaluation of the nutritional importance of proximal and distal small intestine. Ann Surg 1954;140(3):439–48.
15. Mason EE, Ito C. Gastric bypass in obesity. Surg Clin North Am 1967;47(6): 1345–51.
16. Kissileff HR, Nakashima RK, Stunkard AJ. Effects of jejunoileal bypass on meal patterns in genetically obese and lean rats. Am J Physiol 1979;237(3):R217–24.
17. Benfield JR, Greenway FL, Bray GA, et al. Experience with jejunoileal bypass for obesity. Surg Gynecol Obstet 1976;143(3):401–10.
18. Munzberg H, Laque A, Yu S, et al. Appetite and body weight regulation after bariatric surgery. Obes Rev 2015;16(Suppl 1):77–90.
19. Lean ME, Malkova D. Altered gut and adipose tissue hormones in overweight and obese individuals: cause or consequence? Int J Obes (Lond) 2016;40(4):622–32.
20. Chambers AP, Sandoval DA, Seeley RJ. Integration of satiety signals by the central nervous system. Curr Biol 2013;23(9):R379–88.
21. Stefater MA, Wilson-Perez HE, Chambers AP, et al. All bariatric surgeries are not created equal: insights from mechanistic comparisons. Endocr Rev 2012;33(4): 595–622.
22. Stefater MA, Perez-Tilve D, Chambers AP, et al. Sleeve gastrectomy induces loss of weight and fat mass in obese rats, but does not affect leptin sensitivity. Gastroenterology 2010;138(7):2426–36.e1-3.

23. Santulli P, Mandelbrot L, Facchiano E, et al. Obstetrical and neonatal outcomes of pregnancies following gastric bypass surgery: a retrospective cohort study in a French referral centre. Obes Surg 2010;20(11):1501–8.
24. Chagas C, Saunders C, Pereira S, et al. Perinatal outcomes and the influence of maternal characteristics after Roux-en-Y gastric bypass surgery. J Womens Health (Larchmt) 2017;26(1):71–5.
25. Pories WJ, Swanson MS, MacDonald KG, et al. Who would have thought it? An operation proves to be the most effective therapy for adult-onset diabetes mellitus. Ann Surg 1995;222(3):339–50 [discussion: 350–2].
26. Rubino F, Nathan DM, Eckel RH, et al. Metabolic surgery in the treatment algorithm for type 2 diabetes: a joint statement by international diabetes organizations. Diab Care 2016;39(6):861–77.
27. Purnell JQ, Selzer F, Wahed AS, et al. Type 2 diabetes remission rates after laparoscopic gastric bypass and gastric banding: results of the longitudinal assessment of bariatric surgery study. Diabetes care 2016;39(7):1101–7.
28. Jackness C, Karmally W, Febres G, et al. Very low-calorie diet mimics the early beneficial effect of Roux-en-Y gastric bypass on insulin sensitivity and beta-cell function in type 2 diabetic patients. Diabetes 2013;62(9):3027–32.
29. Lingvay I, Guth E, Islam A, et al. Rapid improvement in diabetes after gastric bypass surgery: is it the diet or surgery? Diabetes care 2013;36(9):2741–7.
30. Stylopoulos N, Hoppin AG, Kaplan LM. Roux-en-Y gastric bypass enhances energy expenditure and extends lifespan in diet-induced obese rats. Obesity (Silver Spring) 2009;17(10):1839–47.
31. Dirksen C, Hansen DL, Madsbad S, et al. Postprandial diabetic glucose tolerance is normalized by gastric bypass feeding as opposed to gastric feeding and is associated with exaggerated GLP-1 secretion: a case report. Diabetes care 2010;33(2):375–7.
32. Cohen RV, Schiavon CA, Pinheiro JS, et al. Duodenal-jejunal bypass for the treatment of type 2 diabetes in patients with body mass index of 22-34 kg/m^2: a report of 2 cases. Surg Obes Relat Dis 2007;3(2):195–7.
33. Rajagopalan H, Cherrington AD, Thompson CC, et al. Endoscopic duodenal mucosal resurfacing for the treatment of type 2 diabetes: 6-month interim analysis from the first-in-human proof-of-concept study. Diabetes care 2016;39(12):2254–61.
34. Koehestanie P, de Jonge C, Berends FJ, et al. The effect of the endoscopic duodenal-jejunal bypass liner on obesity and type 2 diabetes mellitus, a multicenter randomized controlled trial. Ann Surg 2014;260(6):984–92.
35. Munoz R, Carmody JS, Stylopoulos N, et al. Isolated duodenal exclusion increases energy expenditure and improves glucose homeostasis in diet-induced obese rats. Am J Physiol Regul Integr Comp Physiol 2012;303(10):R985–93.
36. Adami GF, Cordera R, Marinari G, et al. Plasma ghrelin concentratin in the short-term following biliopancreatic diversion. Obes Surg 2003;13(6):889–92.
37. Karamanakos SN, Vagenas K, Kalfarentzos F, et al. Weight loss, appetite suppression, and changes in fasting and postprandial ghrelin and peptide-YY levels after Roux-en-Y gastric bypass and sleeve gastrectomy: a prospective, double blind study. Ann Surg 2008;247(3):401–7.
38. Morinigo R, Moize V, Musri M, et al. Glucagon-like peptide-1, peptide YY, hunger, and satiety after gastric bypass surgery in morbidly obese subjects. J Clin Endocrinol Metab 2006;91(5):1735–40.
39. le Roux CW, Bueter M, Theis N, et al. Gastric bypass reduces fat intake and preference. Am J Physiol Regul Integr Comp Physiol 2011;301(4):R1057–66.

40. Ochner CN, Gibson C, Shanik M, et al. Changes in neurohormonal gut peptides following bariatric surgery. Int J Obes (Lond) 2011;35(2):153–66.
41. Cummings DE, Weigle DS, Frayo RS, et al. Plasma ghrelin levels after diet-induced weight loss or gastric bypass surgery. N Engl J Med 2002;346(21): 1623–30.
42. Thomas C, Gioiello A, Noriega L, et al. TGR5-mediated bile acid sensing controls glucose homeostasis. Cell Metab 2009;10(3):167–77.
43. Ye J, Hao Z, Mumphrey MB, et al. GLP-1 receptor signaling is not required for reduced body weight after RYGB in rodents. Am J Physiol Regul Integr Comp Physiol 2014;306(5):R352–62.
44. Mokadem M, Zechner JF, Margolskee RF, et al. Effects of Roux-en-Y gastric bypass on energy and glucose homeostasis are preserved in two mouse models of functional glucagon-like peptide-1 deficiency. Mol Metab 2014;3(2):191–201.
45. Chambers AP, Kirchner H, Wilson-Perez HE, et al. The effects of vertical sleeve gastrectomy in rodents are ghrelin independent. Gastroenterology 2013;144(1): 50–2.e5.
46. Jimenez Jaime T, Leiva Balich L, Barrera Acevedo G, et al. Effect of calorie restriction on energy expenditure in overweight and obese adult women. Nutr Hosp 2015;31(6):2428–36.
47. Faria SL, Faria OP, Buffington C, et al. Energy expenditure before and after Roux-en-Y gastric bypass. Obes Surg 2012;22(9):1450–5.
48. Benedetti G, Mingrone G, Marcoccia S, et al. Body composition and energy expenditure after weight loss following bariatric surgery. J Am Coll Nutr 2000; 19(2):270–4.
49. Van Cauter E, Knutson KL. Sleep and the epidemic of obesity in children and adults. Eur J Endocrinol 2008;159(Suppl 1):S59–66.
50. Patel SR, Hu FB. Short sleep duration and weight gain: a systematic review. Obesity (Silver Spring) 2008;16(3):643–53.
51. Reutrakul S, Van Cauter E. Interactions between sleep, circadian function, and glucose metabolism: implications for risk and severity of diabetes. Ann N Y Acad Sci 2014;1311:151–73.
52. Puttonen S, Viitasalo K, Harma M. The relationship between current and former shift work and the metabolic syndrome. Scand J work Environ Health 2012; 38(4):343–8.
53. Ketchum ES, Morton JM. Disappointing weight loss among shift workers after laparoscopic gastric bypass surgery. Obes Surg 2007;17(5):581–4.
54. Watanabe M, Houten SM, Mataki C, et al. Bile acids induce energy expenditure by promoting intracellular thyroid hormone activation. Nature 2006;439(7075):484–9.
55. Kohli R, Bradley D, Setchell KD, et al. Weight loss induced by Roux-en-Y gastric bypass but not laparoscopic adjustable gastric banding increases circulating bile acids. J Clin Endocrinol Metab 2013;98(4):E708–12.
56. Myronovych A, Kirby M, Ryan KK, et al. Vertical sleeve gastrectomy reduces hepatic steatosis while increasing serum bile acids in a weight-loss-independent manner. Obesity (Silver Spring) 2014;22(2):390–400.
57. Scopinaro N, Adami GF, Marinari GM, et al. Biliopancreatic diversion. World J Surg 1998;22(9):936–46.
58. Ryan KK, Tremaroli V, Clemmensen C, et al. FXR is a molecular target for the effects of vertical sleeve gastrectomy. Nature 2014;509(7499):183–8.
59. Flynn CR, Albaugh VL, Cai S, et al. Bile diversion to the distal small intestine has comparable metabolic benefits to bariatric surgery. Nat Commun 2015;6:7715.

60. Kohli R, Setchell KD, Kirby M, et al. A surgical model in male obese rats uncovers protective effects of bile acids post-bariatric surgery. Endocrinology 2013;154(7): 2341–51.
61. Hur KY, Lee MS. Gut microbiota and metabolic disorders. Diabetes Metab J 2015;39(3):198–203.
62. Tremaroli V, Karlsson F, Werling M, et al. Roux-en-Y gastric bypass and vertical banded gastroplasty induce long-term changes on the human gut microbiome contributing to fat mass regulation. Cell Metab 2015;22(2):228–38.
63. Liou AP, Paziuk M, Luevano JM Jr, et al. Conserved shifts in the gut microbiota due to gastric bypass reduce host weight and adiposity. Sci Transl Med 2013; 5(178):178ra41.
64. Mason EE. Ilial transposition and enteroglucagon/GLP-1 in obesity (and diabetic?) surgery. Obes Surg 1999;9(3):223–8.
65. Sullivan S, Stein R, Jonnalagadda S, et al. Aspiration therapy leads to weight loss in obese subjects: a pilot study. Gastroenterology 2013;145(6):1245–52.e1-5.
66. Gunn AJ, Oklu R. A preliminary observation of weight loss following left gastric artery embolization in humans. J Obes 2014;2014:185349.

Endoscopic Treatments Following Bariatric Surgery

Andrew C. Storm, MD, Christopher C. Thompson, MD, MHES*

KEYWORDS

- Bariatric endoscopy • Therapeutic endoscopy • Weight regain
- Endoscopic surgery • Endoscopic suturing • Gastric bypass
- Surgical complications • Fistula

KEY POINTS

- Weight regain after bariatric surgery is common and can be managed with less invasive endoscopic techniques.
- Endoscopic techniques target structural postoperative changes that are associated with weight regain, most notably dilation of the gastrojejunal anastomosis aperture.
- Purse string suture placement, as well as argon plasma coagulation application to the anastomosis, may result in significant and durable weight loss.
- Various endoscopic approaches may be used to safely and effectively manage complications of bariatric surgery, including ulceration and fistula.

INTRODUCTION

Obesity is a lifelong condition of pandemic proportion that requires long-term multidisciplinary management leading up to and beyond any single intervention. Even after restrictive and metabolic surgeries like a Roux-en-Y gastric bypass (RYGB), patients have the potential to experience significant weight regain, which is why a long-term care team is necessary for management of obesity. An emerging member of this care team is the bariatric endoscopist. The field of endobariatrics includes revision procedures for patients who experience weight regain after bariatric surgery, as well as primary endoscopic procedures for the management of obesity.[1] This field also provides medical management of obesity as well as minimally invasive endoscopic

Disclosure Statement: Dr A.C. Storm is a NIH T32 training grant recipient (T32DK007533-31), which supports his research. Dr C.C. Thompson receives consulting fees from Boston Scientific, Covidien, Valentex, Olympus, and receives grants and consulting fees from USGI Medical, Apollo Endosurgery, Fractyl, GI Dynamics, Spatz, GI Windows, and Aspire Bariatrics.
Division of Gastroenterology, Hepatology and Endoscopy, Brigham and Women's Hospital, Harvard Medical School, 75 Francis Street, Boston, MA 02215, USA
* Corresponding author.
E-mail address: cthompson@bwh.harvard.edu

Gastrointest Endoscopy Clin N Am 27 (2017) 233–244
http://dx.doi.org/10.1016/j.giec.2016.12.007
1052-5157/17/© 2017 Elsevier Inc. All rights reserved.

treatments for various complications of bariatric surgery including perforations, leaks, stenosis, and fistulas, to name a few. This article focuses on the currently available endoscopic revision procedures for patients who experience weight regain after bariatric surgery, and also touches on endoscopic techniques in the management of other complications of bariatric surgery that may contribute to weight regain including ulcerations and fistulae.

PATIENT EVALUATION FOR WEIGHT REGAIN AFTER BARIATRIC SURGERY

Prior to offering endoscopic revision procedures, an appropriate infrastructure must be in place. As a part of a multidisciplinary center offering care to the bariatric patient, the customary endoscopy suite will need to make some adjustments to provide safe, dignified, and high-quality care for this patient population. Common adaptations needed to safely and comfortably accommodate bariatric patients include:

- Bariatric specialty furniture for the clinic and endoscopy suite including the waiting areas
- Appropriately sized bathrooms, reinforced toilets and room structure including larger doorways
- Bariatric-rated stretchers and tables for the procedural arena
- Anesthesia team attuned to and comfortable with bariatric patients

As part of the evaluation of the patient with weight regain after bariatric surgery, it is important to obtain a thorough medical history and physical examination. Comorbid conditions that may increase risk associated with procedural sedation are noted, especially because some endoscopic techniques may be safely performed with only conscious sedation, reducing the cost and time required by monitored anesthesiologist care. Prior operative reports should be reviewed to determine the patient's surgical anatomy including any postoperative complications that may have occurred and that will aid in endoscopic procedural planning. The patient's presurgical weight, postsurgical nadir weight, and total weight regained should be recorded. It is important to discuss lifestyle issues related to weight regain, including diet and exercise habits, to determine other contributing factors to the patient's weight regain. In particular, dietary habits to avoid include grazing, rather than eating discrete meals at defined times and consumption of soft calories or sliders, rather than solid whole foods that require chewing and digestion. These 2 eating habits must be addressed prior to consideration of any endoscopic therapy. Appropriate referrals to a dietician, lifestyle coach, and/or psychologist should be made depending on the individual patient.

The cause of weight regain after bariatric surgery is generally multifactorial, but in some cases, reversible medical causes may be at play. Evaluation for medical conditions contributing to weight regain after gastric bypass include:

- Iron studies—Iron deficiency anemia must be corrected
- TSH and free T4—hypothyroidism and other relevant endocrinopathies should be addressed
- Exercise and physical therapy—movement limitations including arthritis should be addressed if possible

Most patients with unresolved obesity, or those who have redeveloped obesity (BMI >30 kg/m^2) and have had all of the previously listed issues addressed should be considered candidates for endoscopic therapy. This is especially true with the presence of comorbid conditions related to obesity (ie, diabetes, hypertension, hyperlipidemia, fatty liver disease, obstructive sleep apnea, or arthritis).

ENDOSCOPIC BARIATRIC REVISION PROCEDURES

Currently available endoscopic techniques for weight loss in the postbariatric surgery patient are primarily aimed at patients who have undergone RYGB, and less commonly those with laparoscopic sleeve gastrectomy (LSG) anatomy. Cumulative numbers of patients who have undergone RYGB in the United States are steadily increasing. Up to 20% of these patients fail to achieve therapeutic success, defined as 50% excess weight loss at 1 year, and another 30% of patients will experience some degree of weight regain, which has no consensus definition, but may be defined as 15% increase from nadir weight.[2–4] This phenomenon of weight regain can affect patient quality of life, lead to return or worsening of comorbid medical conditions, and increases health care expenditure. Although maladaptive eating behaviors and sedentary lifestyle may contribute to weight regain, some reversible structural issues related to the patient's pouch and anatomy also contribute. Surgical revision, including limb-lengthening procedures, are effective and used in up to 13% of RYGB patients with weight regain. However, these are associated with complication rates of up to 50% and mortality rates more than double that of the original surgery, likely owing to the complexity of the non-native abdominal cavity with associated scars, adhesions, and altered anatomy.[5–8] Out of this landscape, minimally invasive endoscopic methods of revision for weight regain after surgical bypass have emerged, targeting the dilated gastric pouch and gastrojejunal anastomosis through use of electrocautery and/or endoscopic suturing or plication techniques.

One landmark study has shown that dilation of the aperture of the gastrojejunal anastomosis (GJA) after surgery is correlated with weight regain after RYGB.[9] In a multivariable logistic regression model, enlarged stomal size was the single greatest predictor of weight regain, and a linear relationship between stomal aperture and weight regain was revealed. Based on these data, stomal diameter greater than or equal to 15 mm may be defined as dilated, and endoscopic revision of the anastomosis should be considered.

Argon Plasma Coagulation

Given the association between dilated GJA and weight regain after RYGB, techniques to reduce the outlet diameter through formation of scar tissue was originally studied using sclerotherapy and more recently through application of argon plasma coagulation (APC).[10–12] Endoscopic sclerotherapy, similar to sclerotherapy of esophageal varices, was accomplished using submucosal needle injection of sodium morrhuate around the gastrojejunal GJA to create edema, scarring, and ideally reduction in aperture of the anastomosis. Because of safety concerns and decreasing availability of sodium morrhuate, as well as the availability of a safer and more easily applied technique using APC, sclerotherapy is no longer utilized. A study of 28 patients receiving sclerotherapy demonstrated that the majority (64%) of patients lost more than 75% of their regained weight after an average 2.3 procedures repeated every 3 to 6 months apart. Anastomotic diameters greater than 15 mm are less likely to benefit from this technique and may benefit more from an endoscopic suturing revision procedure. A similar but newer and safer technique utilizing APC has gained popularity over sclerotherapy.[13,14] In this technique, APC resurfacing of the GJA is accomplished through application of cautery to the gastric side of the anastomosis by touching the tip of a straight-fire APC catheter to the target area. Unlike with most APC techniques, contact with the mucosa is made intentionally to allow for deeper submucosal cautery. This creates a focal coagulation injury to the mucosa as well as the deeper submucosal layers. In 1 study of 30 patients who underwent 3 sessions of APC for weight regain of average 43.2 lbs after their RYGB, an average of 34 lbs were lost. The stomal diameter was reduced 66.9% after completion of these 3 sessions. The authors use pulsed APC with settings of flow 0.8 L/s, effect 2 and 55W. Circumferential resurfacing therapy is applied around the anastomosis in 2 to 3 rings of focal coagulation (**Fig. 1**). Edema, ulceration, and scar tissue formation result in gradual aperture reduction. To allow for maximal healing and to prevent bleeding ulceration, patients are maintained on a twice-daily proton pump inhibitor (PPI), as well as a liquid diet for 45 days after the procedure. Patients typically return for repeat therapy every 8 to 10 weeks for 3 to 4 sessions until the desired aperture size and satiety effect is reached. One international prospective nonrandomized study of 30 patients using APC at 90W revealed that after 3 treatment sessions every 8 weeks, an average 15.5 kg of the average 19 kg regained after bariatric surgery were lost.[14]

The Transoral Outlet Reduction and Purse String

Using the OverStitch platform (Apollo Endosurgery, Austin, Texas) the Transoral Outlet Reduction, or TORe procedure, is used internationally and at many centers across the United States to reduce the aperture of the GJA through use of a purse string suture of the anastomosis. The OverStitch device (**Fig. 2**) is attached to the distal end of a double-channel therapeutic endoscope, which allows for both use of the catheter-based actuating needle for driving and reloading suture, as well as deployment of a helix device to allow for tissue retraction and deeper suture placement.

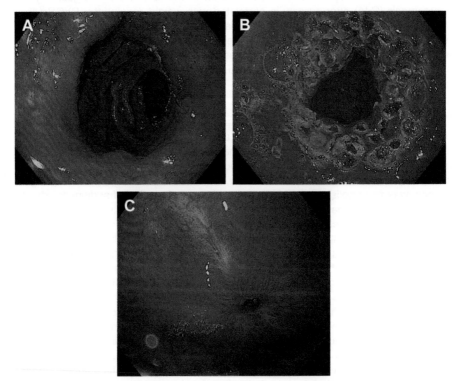

Fig. 1. APC (argon plasma coagulation) resurfacing of the GJA. (*A*) Dilated GJA with aperture of approximately 15 mm. (*B*) APC treatment applied to the gastric side of the stoma. (*C*) In rare cases, overtreatment may result in stenosis requiring dilation.

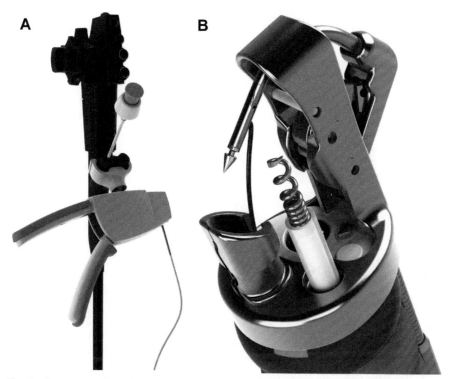

Fig. 2. The OverStitch endoscopic suturing device. (*A*) Handle to drive the needle and needle exchange catheter are attached to a double channel therapeutic endoscope. (*B*) The distal attachment with needle and suture attached to the needle driver arm with helical tissue grabbing tool through the second working channel. (*Courtesy of* Apollo Endosurgery, Incorporated, Austin, TX; with permission.)

For the TORe procedure, an esophageal overtube is placed to protect the proximal esophagus from trauma that may occur with repeated intubations of the suturing device, as it may be removed and replaced through the esophagus during the procedure. To prepare the outlet for suturing, the gastric mucosa adjacent to the anastomosis is treated with APC (forced coagulation, 0.8 L/min, 30 W), and then full-thickness sutures are placed with the needle driven from the jejunal to gastric side of the anastomosis to reduce the aperture (**Fig. 3**). One study of TORe that included 25 patients with dilated GJA resulted, on average, in an aperture reduction from 26.4 mm to 6 mm, with weight loss of 11.7 kg (69.5% of the regained weight was lost) at 6 months without adverse events.[15] In this study, smaller apertures resulted in increased nausea and vomiting and higher stitch loss with subsequent weight loss failure. As such, a modified technique using a purse string suture pattern was developed. Depending on the size of the outlet, 8 to 12 running stitches are placed using a single suture to create a purse string. Upon completion of the purse string, the suture is tightened over an 8 mm through-the-scope esophageal balloon to size the final outlet diameter.

A randomized, sham-controlled, multicenter trial of transoral outlet reduction using the Bard Endocinch device (CR Bard, Inc. Murray Hill, NJ, USA) was completed, and provided level 1 evidence for the short-term safety and efficacy of TORe.[16] In this study, patients who underwent TORe experienced significantly greater weight loss than controls (3.5% vs 0.4%, *P* = .21). Systolic blood pressure was statistically

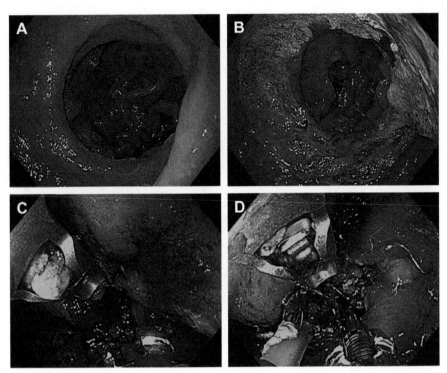

Fig. 3. The TORe (transoral outlet revision) procedure. (*A*) Dilated stoma of approximately 25 mm is examined. (*B*) APC cautery is applied to the gastric musoca around the stoma. (*C*) Full-thickness purse-string suture is then placed around the stoma. (*D*) Final aperture is sized using an 8 mm balloon.

improved, and there was a trend toward improved metabolic parameters. This TORe study was performed with the EndoCinch suction-based superficial mucosal suturing device. Newer devices, as with the Apollo OverStitch, allow for full-thickness suturing and improved durability. A study comparing outlet reduction using the full-thickness OverStitch device to the superficial suturing with the EndoCinch device in 118 patients revealed superior weight loss in the OverStitch patients at both 6 and 12 months.[17] A follow-up study showed enhanced durability with this system at 3 years, with an average 19.2% excess weight loss at the 3-year mark after TORe.[18] This summarizes the most complete body of work regarding revision of gastric bypass, showing the procedure's effectiveness and durability within a multidisciplinary plan of care.

Postprocedure recommendations after completion of TORe include

1. Twice-daily PPI (ie, omeprazole 40 mg opened into applesauce) for 6 weeks
2. Staged diet: 48 hours clear liquids, 6 weeks full liquid diet, 2 weeks of soft solid foods followed by a solid calorie diet for maintenance

The Incisionless Operating Platform, or IOP (USGI, San Clemente, California) used in the Primary Obesity Surgery, Endolumenal (POSE) procedure, has also been studied for endoscopic revision and management of weight regain after RYGB termed the Revision Obesity Surgery, Endolumenal, or ROSE procedure (**Fig. 4**). Specifically, this procedure is considered for patients with weight regain in the setting of an enlarged pouch as well as a dilated GJA. Full-thickness plications are placed with

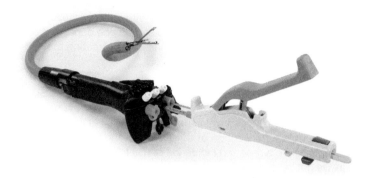

Fig. 4. The IOP (Incisionless Operating Platform). This disposable 1-time use platform employs use of a slim gastroscope through 1 channel for visualization (not shown), and includes a tissue plication device (shown) through the main operating channel. (*Courtesy of USGI, San Clemente, CA; with permission.*)

the disposable transoral platform with the goal of reducing both pouch size and anastomosis aperture. A study of 20 patients undergoing ROSE demonstrated technical success in 85% of patients, with weight loss of 8.8 kg at 3 months.[19] This study emphasized the importance of revising both the outlet and pouch, rather than the pouch alone. Particularly important to successful weight loss was reduction of the GJA to less than 1 cm. A larger prospective multicenter study of 116 patients achieved technical success in 97% of patients, with 32% of the weight regained after RYGB lost at 6 months and no significant adverse events.[20]

Other techniques of outlet revision have been reported; however, these are limited to small series, and mainstream adoption have not occurred. One technique used to address the pouch and GJA dilation includes use of a large over-the-scope clip to reduce the rapid emptying that may occur with stomal dilation.[21] Another technique, using radiofrequency ablation to treat the pouch and stoma in 25 patients reported 18.4% excess weight loss at 12 months.[22] Reduction of the pouch and outlet using varied fasteners has also been reported, but these fasteners not commonly used today.[23]

Weight Regain after Sleeve Gastrectomy

Patients who have previously undergone LSG may regain weight if the sleeve is dilated from food bolus consumption over time. As in the case of a dilated RYGB pouch, the dilated sleeve may be managed with endoscopic suturing or tissue plication to reduce the sleeve diameter. Several reports exist detailing the feasibility and safety of this revision procedure using endoscopic suturing to reduce the sleeve volume; however, more data will needed before this can be considered for mainstream use.[24]

ENDOSCOPIC MANAGEMENT OF OTHER COMPLICATIONS OF BARIATRIC SURGERY

Other complications of bariatric surgery may be implicated in weight regain. Gastrogastric fistula formation essentially results in metabolic reversal of an RYGB, as foodstuff may be permitted to enter the remnant stomach, which may (1) serve as a reservoir for increased volume of consumption and (2) will negate the metabolic effects of the bypass surgery, allowing nutrient intake to be exposed to and absorbed by the previously excluded duodenum and proximal jejunum. Marginal ulceration, which may lead to iron deficiency anemia, is also often diagnosed and managed by the endoscopist. Marginal ulceration may lead to pain with eating, resulting in conversion to soft calories. Both iron deficiency anemia and soft calorie consumption have been associated with weight regain. Endoscopic techniques for treating these 2 conditions will be reviewed.

Gastro-Gastric Fistula

Gastro-gastric fistula formation was a common complication of the nondivided RYGB surgical technique, previously reported in up to nearly 50% of cases.[25] Over the past decade, routine complete transection of the stomach and gastric pouch has significantly reduced this risk to a reported incidence of 0% to 6%.[26] Gastro-gastric fistulae often result in weight regain due to nutrients entering the gastric remnant and duodenum with reversal of the metabolic effects of the RYGB. In rare cases, complete reversal of the bypass anatomy may occur with stenosis of the GJA due to recurrent ulceration and dilation of the fistula. Endoscopic therapies for gastro-gastric fistulae, including clips, glue, and endoscopic suturing have been reported and are increasingly considered as the first-line approach given the substantial morbidity and mortality associated with repeat surgery. Although the availability of various endoscopic approaches will depend on a center's expertise, endoscopic suturing of the fistula has been studied with the most success in durable fistula closure (**Fig. 5**); however,

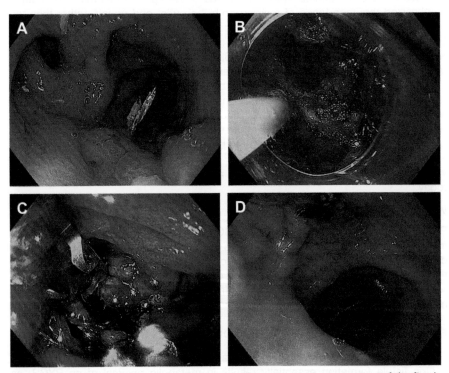

Fig. 5. Closure of a gastro-gastric fistula through ESD and endoscopic suturing of the fistula. (*A*) The fistula is shown here to the left of the GJA. (*B*) ESD is performed around the fistula opening to expose the muscular layer and then APC used to ablate any remaining mucosa. (*C*) Running suture placed to close the defect. (*D*) Fistula now fully closed on final inspection.

results are still limited. An initial study of 95 patients undergoing endoscopic gastro-gastric fistula closure demonstrated initial success in 95% of patients, although 65% of patients had recurrent fistula.[27] In this study, the only significant predictor of fistula recurrence was an initial fistula diameter greater than 20 mm. A multicenter study of 20 patients using the OverStitch device achieved immediate closure in 100% of patients, with long-term closure in 6 patients (30%).[28] Another study reported durable endoscopic closure in 4 out of 6 patients (66.7%) with gastro-gastric fistula, suggesting that a subset of patients with gastro-gastric fistula may be best managed with endoscopic therapy, although more research on the ideal technique and patient selection is needed.[29]

Marginal Ulceration and Bleeding

Marginal ulcerations may occur in up to 16% of patients after gastric bypass as a result of suture material, large gastric pouch, diabetes, use of tobacco cigarettes or *Helicobacter pylori* infection, among other causes.[30] Ulceration may result in either weight loss because of postprandial pain, or paradoxically may result in weight gain through the mechanism of transitioning the diet to soft foods and liquids, which allows for increased calorie intake. Ulcerations may also result in occult blood loss and iron deficiency anemia, which can lead to appetite stimulation with weight gain and may also lead to perforation and peritonitis requiring emergency surgery with high mortality risk. As such, healing any ulcer(s) is of paramount importance to the patient. If the patient smokes tobacco, cessation counseling and pharmacotherapy aimed at cessation should be offered. Nonsteroidal anti-inflammatory drug (NSAID) medications should also be discontinued if possible. Additionally, the authors recommend the following aggressive medical therapy

1. High-dose PPI (ie, omeprazole 40 mg) twice daily 15 to 30 minutes before meals, opening the capsule into apple sauce
2. Sucralfate 1 g up to 4 times daily 1 hour after meals to coat the ulcer and promote healing of the ulcer—these medications should be opened or crushed, respectively, or supplied in liquid form to ensure absorption and efficacy of the medications

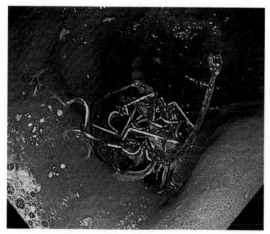

Fig. 6. Extruded suture and staple material at the GJA. This may lead to ulcers, pain, and intermittent partial obstruction when foodstuff becomes impacted and tangled in the suture material.

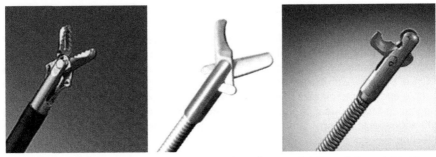

Fig. 7. Tools used for removal of the suture and staple material. From left to right: biopsy forceps, reusable scissors, and loop cutters. (*Courtesy of* Olympus America, Waltham, MA; with permission.)

Some research shows that marginal ulceration will not heal as effectively without opening the PPI capsule or taking soluble formulation; as such the PPI and sucralfate must be opened, crushed, or supplied in suspension.[31] Alterations in gastrointestinal pH, blood flow, and absorptive surface area have been previously implicated in altered pharmaceutical concentrations after gastric bypass.[32]

If foreign material (suture or staples) from the prior surgery is present at the site of ulceration (**Fig. 6**), the authors routinely remove this endoscopically to promote healing.[33] Tools including endoscopic scissors, loop cutters, and simple biopsy forceps may be used to cut or tear the protruding suture material (**Fig. 7**). Loop cutters may jam when used to cut braided or silk suture and should be used only for monofilament for this reason.

In the case of a bleeding ulcer, a standard approach using the Forrest classification should be taken, with care to avoid perforation of this weakened, sometimes ischemic area near or upon the surgical anastomosis site.[34] For active bleeding and visible vessel, dual endoscopic therapy with epinephrine injection and mechanical hemostasis (hemoclip placement) is advised, as with any gastric ulcer. In rare cases, nonhealing ulcers have been managed with endoscopic oversewing with advancement of a mucosal flap using the OverStitch device.[35] Reoperation and surgical revision are reserved for the most recalcitrant ulcers.[36]

SUMMARY/DISCUSSION

The prevalence and societal cost of obesity and its complications have made it a primary public health concern. Surgical approaches to weight loss are effective, but fall short in achieving complete and long-term weight loss for some patients. As in other medical subspecialties like interventional cardiology and pulmonology, less invasive intraluminal endoscopic approaches are being developed to address the significant cost and morbidity associated with similar but more invasive surgical techniques. Endoscopic transoral outlet reduction of the GJA is the only bariatric revision procedure with level 1 evidence to support its use. In the obese patient population, endobariatric techniques aiming to reduce the diameter of the GJA and pouch size in patients with prior RYGB, and sleeve diameter in patients with LSG, are safe and effective options that are becoming increasingly available. Similarly, many complications of bariatric surgical procedures, including ulceration and gastro-gastric fistula, which may contribute to weight regain, may be managed safely and effectively through the endoscopic approach.

Key to the success of these techniques, as with any modality targeting weight loss, is that they exist within a multidisciplinary approach. Gastroenterologists and other skilled endoscopists add a large number of physicians to the pool required to meet the demand of managing the obesity pandemic. Societies and organizations must continue working together to champion code development and reimbursement to increase availability of these and other emerging therapies.

REFERENCES

1. ASGE Bariatric Endoscopy Task Force, ASGE Technology Committee, Abu Dayyeh BK, et al. Endoscopic bariatric therapies. Gastrointest Endosc 2015; 81(5):1073–86.
2. Brolin RE. Bariatric surgery and long-term control of morbid obesity. JAMA 2002; 288(22):2793–6.
3. McCormick JT, Papasavas PK, Caushaj PF, et al. Laparoscopic revision of failed open bariatric procedures. Surg Endosc 2003;17(3):413–5.
4. Powers PS, Rosemurgy A, Boyd F, et al. Outcome of gastric restriction procedures: weight, psychiatric diagnoses, and satisfaction. Obes Surg 1997;7(6):471–7.
5. Behrns KE, Smith CD, Kelly KA, et al. Reoperative bariatric surgery. Lessons learned to improve patient selection and results. Ann Surg 1993;218(5):646–53.
6. Coakley BA, Deveney CW, Spight DH, et al. Revisional bariatric surgery for failed restrictive procedures. Surg Obes Relat Dis 2008;4(5):581–6.
7. Linner JH, Drew RL. Reoperative surgery—indications, efficacy, and long-term follow-up. Am J Clin Nutr 1992;55(2 Suppl):606S–10S.
8. Buchwald H, Estok R, Fahrbach K, et al. Trends in mortality in bariatric surgery: a systematic review and meta-analysis. Surgery 2007;142(4):621–32 [discussion: 32–5].
9. Abu Dayyeh BK, Lautz DB, Thompson CC. Gastrojejunal stoma diameter predicts weight regain after Roux-en-Y gastric bypass. Clin Gastroenterol Hepatol 2011; 9(3):228–33.
10. Thompson CC, Slattery J, Bundga ME, et al. Peroral endoscopic reduction of dilated gastrojejunal anastomosis after Roux-en-Y gastric bypass: a possible new option for patients with weight regain. Surg Endosc 2006;20(11):1744–8.
11. Spaulding L, Osler T, Patlak J. Long-term results of sclerotherapy for dilated gastrojejunostomy after gastric bypass. Surg Obes Relat Dis 2007;3(6):623–6.
12. Abidi WM, Schulman A, Thompson CC. 1137 A large case series on the use of argon plasma coagulation for the treatment of weight regain after gastric bypass. Gastroenterology 2016;150(4):S231.
13. Aly A. Argon plasma coagulation and gastric bypass—a novel solution to stomal dilation. Obes Surg 2009;19(6):788–90.
14. Baretta GA, Alhinho HC, Matias JE, et al. Argon plasma coagulation of gastrojejunal anastomosis for weight regain after gastric bypass. Obes Surg 2015;25(1):72–9.
15. Jirapinyo P, Slattery J, Ryan MB, et al. Evaluation of an endoscopic suturing device for transoral outlet reduction in patients with weight regain following Roux-en-Y gastric bypass. Endoscopy 2013;45(7):532–6.
16. Thompson CC, Chand B, Chen YK, et al. Endoscopic suturing for transoral outlet reduction increases weight loss after Roux-en-Y gastric bypass surgery. Gastroenterology 2013;145(1):129–37.e3.
17. Kumar N, Thompson CC. Comparison of a superficial suturing device with a full-thickness suturing device for transoral outlet reduction (with videos). Gastrointest Endosc 2014;79(6):984–9.
18. Kumar N, Thompson CC. Transoral outlet reduction for weight regain after gastric bypass: long-term follow-up. Gastrointest Endosc 2016;83(4):776–9.

19. Mullady DK, Lautz DB, Thompson CC. Treatment of weight regain after gastric bypass surgery when using a new endoscopic platform: initial experience and early outcomes (with video). Gastrointest Endosc 2009;70(3):440–4.

20. Horgan S, Jacobsen G, Weiss GD, et al. Incisionless revision of post-Roux-en-Y bypass stomal and pouch dilation: multicenter registry results. Surg Obes Relat Dis 2010;6(3):290–5.

21. Heylen AM, Jacobs A, Lybeer M, et al. The OTSC(R)-clip in revisional endoscopy against weight gain after bariatric gastric bypass surgery. Obes Surg 2011; 21(10):1629–33.

22. Abrams J, Komanduri S, Shaheen N, et al. Mo1947 radiofrequency ablation for the treatment of weight regain after roux-en-Y gastric bypass surgery. Gastroenterology 2016;150(4):S824.

23. Eid GM, McCloskey CA, Eagleton JK, et al. StomaphyX vs a sham procedure for revisional surgery to reduce regained weight in Roux-en-Y gastric bypass patients: a randomized clinical trial. JAMA Surg 2014;149(4):372–9.

24. Sharaiha RZ, Kedia P, Kumta N, et al. Endoscopic sleeve plication for revision of sleeve gastrectomy. Gastrointest Endosc 2015;81(4):1004.

25. Capella JF, Capella RF. Gastro-gastric fistulas and marginal ulcers in gastric bypass procedures for weight reduction. Obes Surg 1999;9(1):22–7 [discussion: 8].

26. Carrodeguas L, Szomstein S, Soto F, et al. Management of gastrogastric fistulas after divided Roux-en-Y gastric bypass surgery for morbid obesity: analysis of 1,292 consecutive patients and review of literature. Surg Obes Relat Dis 2005;1(5):467–74.

27. Fernandez-Esparrach G, Lautz DB, Thompson CC. Endoscopic repair of gastro-gastric fistula after Roux-en-Y gastric bypass: a less-invasive approach. Surg Obes Relat Dis 2010;6(3):282–8.

28. Mukewar S, Kumar N, Catalano M, et al. Safety and efficacy of fistula closure by endoscopic suturing: a multi-center study. Endoscopy 2016;48(11):1023–8.

29. Campos JN, Galvão M, Martins J, et al. Endoscopic, conservative, and surgical treatment of the gastrogastric fistula: the efficacy of a stepwise approach and its long-term results. Bariatric Surg Pract Patient Care 2015;10(2):62–7.

30. Azagury DE, Abu Dayyeh BK, Greenwalt IT, et al. Marginal ulceration after Roux-en-Y gastric bypass surgery: characteristics, risk factors, treatment, and outcomes. Endoscopy 2011;43(11):950–4.

31. Schulman A, Devery A, Thompson CC. Su1060 opening PPI capsules should be the new standard of care in the treatment of marginal ulceration. Gastrointest Endosc 2016;83(5):AB314.

32. Benet LZKD, Sheiner LB. Pharmacokinetics: the dynamics of drug absorption, distribution and elimination. In: Hardman JG, Limbird LE, editors. Goodman and Gilman's the pharmacological basis of therapeutics. 9th edition. New York: McGraw-Hill; 1996. p. 3–27.

33. Lee JK, Van Dam J, Morton JM, et al. Endoscopy is accurate, safe, and effective in the assessment and management of complications following gastric bypass surgery. Am J Gastroenterol 2009;104(3):575–82 [quiz: 83].

34. Forrest JA, Finlayson ND, Shearman DJ. Endoscopy in gastrointestinal bleeding. Lancet 1974;2(7877):394–7.

35. Jirapinyo P, Watson RR, Thompson CC. Use of a novel endoscopic suturing device to treat recalcitrant marginal ulceration (with video). Gastrointest Endosc 2012;76(2):435–9.

36. Fringeli Y, Worreth M, Langer I. Gastrojejunal anastomosis complications and their management after laparoscopic Roux-en-Y Gastric bypass. J Obes 2015; 2015:698425.

Intragastric Balloons in Clinical Practice

Marianna Papademetriou, MD[a], Violeta Popov, MD, PhD[b],*

KEYWORDS

- Intragastric balloons • Obesity • Weight loss • Review • Efficacy

KEY POINTS

- Intragastric balloons (IGBs) are a minimally invasive endoscopic weight loss method available for use in the United States.
- IGBs consistently lead to 10% to 15% total body weight loss and improvement in metabolic risk factors, with a low rate of serious adverse events.
- The most common adverse events are postimplantation nausea and vomiting, and early removal of the device owing to intolerance.
- Effective early management of symptoms can prevent or reduce these complications.
- Successful use in practice requires a multidisciplinary approach and long-term follow-up plan.

The current standard of care for weight loss is caloric restriction with dietary changes and increased calorie expenditure through exercise. Should this strategy prove insufficient or lack durability, medical therapy can be added. Many patients continue to struggle with weight loss and may then consider more invasive approaches. Bariatric surgery provides the most effective and durable method of weight loss. However, bariatric surgery is associated with mortality in 0.2% to 1.0% of cases, a reoperation rate of 4.3% to 8.3%, and serious adverse events in 26%.[1] Furthermore, many patients in various parts of the United States do not have access to comprehensive bariatric surgery centers.[2] Owing to concern over potential complications as well as lack of availability, only a small percentage of obese patients require and qualify for bariatric surgery to treat obesity and associated metabolic conditions.[3] Thus, novel treatment strategies that are more effective than diet and pharmacotherapy and safer than surgery are being developed.

Disclosure Statement: The authors have nothing to disclose.
[a] Gastroenterology, New York University School of Medicine, 220 First Avenue, New York, NY 10016, USA; [b] Division of Gastroenterology, NY VA Harbor Healthcare (Manhattan), New York University School of Medicine, 423 East 23rd Street, 15 North, New York, NY 10010, USA
* Corresponding author.
E-mail address: Violeta.popov@nyumc.org

Gastrointest Endoscopy Clin N Am 27 (2017) 245–256
http://dx.doi.org/10.1016/j.giec.2016.12.006
1052-5157/17/Published by Elsevier Inc.

giendo.theclinics.com

INTRAGASTRIC BALLOONS

Intragastric balloon (IGB) devices are the most popular minimally invasive option for treatment of obesity. Early devices released in the 1980s, however, were ineffective and potentially hazardous. The first such device was the Garren-Edwards Gastric Bubble,[4] an air-filled balloon. About 20,000 such devices were implanted. In practice, spontaneous deflation occurred in 31% of cases and gastric ulcers were seen in 26%.[5] Adverse events including gastric perforations and intestinal obstructions requiring surgical extraction eventually led to the withdrawal of the device. Nevertheless, this encouraged the development of safer and more effective IGBs.

The second-generation IGBs have been used outside of the United States for more than 25 years. These balloons are made of more durable silicone-based material and filled with saline or air. The most commonly used IGB worldwide is the Bioenterics Intragastric Balloon, a fluid-filled single balloon, marketed in the United States as the Orbera Intragastric Balloon System (Apollo Endosurgery, Austin, TX). More than 250,000 Orbera balloons have been placed since its introduction in 1996. It was approved for use in the United States in 2015.

ReShape (ReShape Medical Inc., San Clemente, CA), a dual balloon system, was approved at the same time. In September 2016, the US Food and Drug Administration (FDA) approved a gastric balloon that is swallowed, the Obalon (Obalon Therapeutics, San Diego, CA). The Obalon Balloon is unique in that it allows for placement through the swallowing of a deflated balloon in the form of a capsule. Owing to the smaller overall capacity of 250 mL, up to 3 balloons can be placed in the stomach over a 3-month period. The Obalon balloons are filled with nitrogen mixed gas rather than saline through a catheter that remains attached until the balloon is fully inflated within the stomach.[6] All 3 IGBs are approved for patients with a body mass index (BMI) of 30 to 40 kg/m^2 who have failed nutritional counseling and lifestyle therapy. Until recently, there was no other effective weight loss procedure available for this group, because a BMI of 40 kg/m^2 is usually required for consideration of bariatric surgery.

MECHANISM OF ACTION

The mechanism of action by which IGBs lead to weight loss is multifactorial and incompletely understood. It is hypothesized that these devices facilitate weight loss by reducing the stomach's potential volume and inducing early satiety (**Fig. 1**). In this manner, total caloric intake for the day may be reduced with adherence to nutritional counseling. Additional proposed mechanisms include changes in gastric emptying and hormonal changes. One study found that gastric emptying rates are reduced at 1 and 4 months after balloon insertion, and return to normal 1 month after balloon removal. Recent experiments added additional evidence to the role of delayed gastric emptying in promoting weight loss after IGB placement.[7] A subset of patients with normal or increased gastric emptying times before balloon placement experienced greater weight loss with IGB therapy compared with patients with baseline delayed emptying. The group with baseline delayed emptying may benefit from different mechanistic approaches to achieve weight loss other than IGBs.

Other proposed mechanisms include changes in appetite-regulating hormones. Fasting plasma ghrelin and leptin were decreased significantly when the balloon was in the stomach, leading to decreased hunger.[8] However, there are conflicting reports of observed hormonal changes in other studies. It is likely that many of these factors together contribute to the overall weight loss achieved.

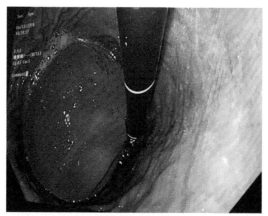

Fig. 1. Placement of an intragastric balloon. (*Courtesy of* Apollo Endosurgery, Inc., Austin, TX; with permission.)

TYPES OF INTRAGASTRIC BALLOONS APPROVED FOR USE IN THE UNITED STATES

1. Obera[9]
    a. Saline-filled single balloon system
    b. Fill volume of 500 to 750 mL
    c. Placed endoscopically
    d. Implanted for up to 6 months
    e. Requires endoscopy for deflation and removal
2. ReShape Duo[10]
    a. Saline-filled double balloon system
    b. Fill volume of 450 mL/balloon for total of 900 mL
    c. Placed endoscopically
    d. Implanted for up to 6 months
    e. Requires endoscopy for deflation and removal
3. Obalon[6]
    a. Gas-filled multiballoon system
    b. Fill volume of 250 mL; up to 3 balloons may be placed
    c. Swallowed capsule delivery device
    d. Does not require endoscopy or sedation for placement; placement in the stomach is confirmed with fluoroscopy before inflation
    e. Implanted for up to 6 months
    f. Requires endoscopy for deflation and removal; all 3 balloons are removed at the same time

WEIGHT LOSS AND METABOLIC OUTCOMES IN INTRAGASTRIC BALLOON TRIALS

IGBs were only recently approved by the FDA in the United States; however, efficacy for achieving weight loss with IGB was established through early trials in Europe. Patients included in these trials were either not candidates for bariatric surgery or refused bariatric surgery. A retrospective study of 2515 patients in Italy, one of the largest to date, showed a mean BMI loss of 4.9 ± 12 kg/m^2 over the 6-month study period. Among obesity-related comorbidities, including hypertension, diabetes, respiratory disorders, dyslipidemia, and osteoarthropathy, 44.3% had resolution and another 44.8% had improvement of conditions over the study period.[11]

Other studies corroborate the effectiveness of IGB for weight loss. Mean excess weight was reduced from 48.5 to 28.5 kg, with reduction in BMI from 44.1 to 38.4 kg/m^2 in 1 study of 231 patients.[12] In a metaanalysis, the pooled mean for excess weight loss was 32.1%, and 12.2% for total body weight loss.[13]

Several randomized, controlled trials have examined the efficacy and effectiveness of IGBs compared with diet and lifestyle therapy (**Table 1**).[11,14–22] One trial compared the effectiveness of IGB with pharmacotherapy: 50 obese patients were assigned randomly to lifestyle modification with IGB placement or lifestyle modification with pharmacotherapy with sibutramine. After balloon removal, patients were again randomly assigned to either lifestyle changes alone, or lifestyle changes plus pharmacotherapy. This study found that, at 12 months, patients within the IGB group with or without sibutramine lost significantly more weight compared with patients who received only pharmacotherapy.[17] The Obalon and Reshape Duo, the 2 other FDA-approved IGBs, have similar efficacy in achieving weight loss.[14,22]

More recent studies have demonstrated not only sustained weight loss effects, but additional health outcomes achieved by IGB placement. In a randomized, controlled study by Fuller and colleagues,[23] 66 obese adults were randomized to IGB and behavioral modification versus behavior modification alone. In this high-quality trial, subjects receiving IGB placement has significantly greater weight loss than the control group, with a mean weight loss of 14.2 kg. This weight loss was associated with a greater reduction in waist circumference and importantly, an improvement in quality of life compared with the control group. Furthermore, the subjects were followed out to 12 months and had sustained weight loss of 9.2 kg compared with 5.2 kg in controls.[23]

A metaanalysis of 10 randomized, controlled trials and 30 observational studies with 5668 patients evaluated the impact of IGBs on metabolic comorbidities. IGBs significantly improved fasting glucose, hemoglobin A1C, triglycerides, blood pressure, and waist circumference. Hemoglobin A1C decreased by 17% and fasting glucose by 15% in patients with diabetes. The odds ratio for achieving diabetes remission was 1.4 (95% confidence interval, 1.3–1.6) at the end of treatment with IGB.[24] Another metaanalysis demonstrated the benefit of IGB in improving liver enzymes and nonalcoholic fatty liver disease in patients with obesity.[25] Thus, IGB therapy may provide an additional treatment option for patients with the metabolic syndrome, as part of a multidisciplinary team approach.

ADVERSE EVENTS

Overall, the frequency of significant complications with IGB therapy seems to be low. The most common adverse events include nausea, vomiting, and decreased oral intake. Many of these symptoms can be managed conservatively without the need for early balloon removal.

In the largest retrospective study to date of 2515 patients with IGB, there were 5 gastric perforations and 2 deaths.[11] Those data, collected from 2000 to 2004, helped to identify prior gastric surgery as an absolute contraindication to gastric balloon placement, because these patients had a higher proportion of complications overall. A randomized, controlled trial from the same investigators did not observe any serious adverse events.[17]

A 2008 meta-analysis of randomized, controlled trials identified an early removal rate of balloons of 4.2%. The majority of these were done for abdominal pain or other mild digestive disorders. Obstruction of the digestive tract was the cause of early removal in 0.6% of patients undergoing early removal, and was overall very rare.[13] In a more recent metaanalysis of 68 observational studies published in 2015, pain

Table 1
Summary of IGB trials and outcomes with serious adverse events

First Author, Year	Country	Balloon Type	Study Type	Implant Time	N cases N controls	Diet/Lifestyle	Initial BMI kg/m² (SD)	BMI Lost (SD)	%EWL	%TBWL	Adverse Events
Ponce et al,[14] 2015	US	Reshape Duo	RCT	6 mo	187 / 139	Hypocaloric diet	35.3 (2.8) / 35.4 (2.6)	2.7 (1.9) / 1.3 (2.3)	27.9 (21.3) / 12.3 (22.1)	7.6 (5.5) / 3.6 (6.3)	NR
Fuller et al,[23] 2013	Australia	Orbera	RCT	6 mo	30 / 20	T2DM Lifestyle diet; 10,000 steps/d	36 (2.7) / 36.7 (2.9)	5.1	50.3	14.2	1 early removal
Genco et al,[11] 2006	Italy	Orbera	RCT	3 mo	16 / 16	1000 kcal/d diet	43.9 (1.1) / 43.6 (1.8)	5.8 (0.5) / 0.4 (0.2)	34 (4.8) / 2.1 (1)	NR	No serious AE
Martinez-Brocca,[15] 2007	Spain	Orbera	RCT	6 mo	11 / 10	Low fat hypocaloric diet	50.2 (9.6) / 51.3 (6.1)	4.5	12.7 kg	12.7	NR
Mathus-Vliegen,[18] 2002	Netherlands	Orbera	RCT	13 wk	20 / 23	1000–1500 kcal/d	43 (1.3) / 43.6 (1.6)	4.6	NR	10.6 (.88)	No serious AE
Mathus-Vliegen,[5] 2014	Netherlands	Orbera	RCT	13 wk	19 / 23	1000–1500 kcal/d	43 (5.5) / 43.2 (7.1)	—	—	—	—
Lee et al,[16] 2012	Singapore	Orbera	RCT	6 mo	11 / 10	1200–1500 kcal/d	43 (5.5) / 43.6 (7.6)	1.52 (0.36–3.3)	NR	NR	NR
Farina et al,[17] 2012	Italy	Orbera	RCT	12 mo	30 / 20	900–1500 kcal/d, 30 min exercise 5 d/wk	42.3 (1) / 41 (1.3)	6.3 (1.2)	NR	17.4 (3.4)	No serious AE
Genco et al,[11] 2005	Italy	Orbera	Case series	6 mo	2515 / —	1000 kcal/d diet	44.4 (7.8) / —	4.9 (12.7)	33.9	NR	5 (0.19%) perforations 2 deaths
Machytka et al,[19] 2011	Czech Republic	Spatz	Pilot	12 mo	18 / —	1000 kcal/d diet	37.3	NR	48.8	NR	5 early removals 2 device leaks
Brooks,[29] 2014	UK	Spatz	Case series	12 mo	73 / —	1000 kcal/d diet	36.6 (11)	NR	24.8	20.1	3 surgical extractions
Machytka, 2016	Czech Republic	Elipse	Pilot	6 wk	8 / —	No diet	31	NR	12.4	NR	No serious AE
Chittani, 2016	Czech Rep. Greece	Elipse	Case series	16 wk	25 / —	Lifestyle counseling	34.8	3.9	39	10	4 (16%) balloons vomited
Sullivan,[22] 2016	US	Obalon	RCT	6 mo	185 / 181	Lifestyle therapy	35.2 (2.7) / 35.5 (2.7)	NR	NR	6.8 / 3.6	9.6% early removal

Abbreviations: %TBWL, percent total body weight lost; %EWL, percent excess weight lost; AE, adverse event; NR, not reported; RCT, randomized controlled trial; SD, standard deviation; T2DM, type 2 diabetes mellitus.

and nausea were frequent side effects, occurring in 33.7% and 29% of subjects, respectively. The pooled early removal rate was 7.5%. Serious adverse events were infrequent. Migration occurred in 1.4% of cases, small bowel obstruction in 0.3%, and gastric perforation in 0.1% of patients.[26]

INTRAGASTRIC BALLOONS IN CLINICAL PRACTICE

Endoscopically placed IGBs may be initiated at an institution or a private practice setting as part of a comprehensive multidisciplinary weight loss program.

For institutions or practices seeking to begin a comprehensive bariatric program, support from multiple services is needed. In addition to a gastroenterologist trained in bariatric procedures, other services include registered dieticians, life coaches, gastrointestinal endoscopy nurses, and mental health providers, as well as bariatric surgeons. Whether in private practice or academics, the participating medical professionals need to prepare a business plan to help determine costs of a bariatric endoscopy program with IGBs. Such a plan should take into account the cost of placing and removing the balloon, related anesthesia and facility charges, the device itself, and the cost of the aftercare program, as well as training of personnel. Aftercare can be provided by a dietician within the practice, or via an online live coaching program. Finally, the gastroenterologist will need to consider possible complications and how to factor those in the overall cost. A structured algorithm for managing postprocedure symptoms is also recommended.

Appropriate patient selection is critical for success of the procedure itself, as well as successful sustained weight loss after the balloon is removed. Patients should be motivated to lose weight and committed to engaging in lifelong behavior modification before and after placement of the IGB. One of the key predictors of success with weight loss procedures is the frequency and compliance with follow-up.

Expectations should be set with the patient before placement of IGB. Successful durable weight loss using IGB placement relies on behavior modification that is sustainable after device removal. For this reason, IGB placement should be used in conjunction with a long-term supervised diet and behavior modification program to increase likelihood of significant weight loss and maintenance. Currently, the FDA recommends that the patients participate in a lifestyle program for 12 months: 6 months while the balloon is implanted, and another 6 months after the balloon is removed. In our practice, the patients are enrolled for 13 months altogether. Patients meet with the gastroenterologists for preprocedural counseling and assessment, and also see the nutritionist at least twice before the balloon placement (**Fig. 2**). Thereafter, they continue to see the nutritionist on a monthly basis for the duration of the program.

The following inclusion and exclusion criteria are recommended for consideration in patient selection.

Inclusion criteria
- Adults greater than 18 and less than 70 years of age.
- BMI of 30 to 40 kg/m^2
- Failed conventional weight loss therapies including increase physical activity and decrease caloric intake.

IGB absolute contraindications
- Oropharyngeal obstruction or altered anatomy
- Partial or complete esophageal obstruction
- Prior gastric surgery
- Gastric mass

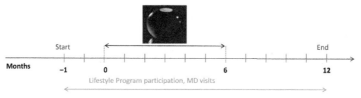

Fig. 2. Setup of a multidisciplinary program with intragastric balloon and lifestyle counseling. (*Courtesy of* Apollo Endosurgery, Inc., Austin, TX; with permission.)

- Large hiatal hernia (>4 cm)
- Presence of esophageal or gastric varices
- Presence of congenital atresias or stenosis in the upper gastrointestinal tract
- Achalasia

Relative exclusion criteria
- History of untreated coronary artery disease or decompensated congestive heart failure
- Anemia
- Unstable thyroid disease
- Chronic use of narcotic pain medication
- Alcohol use of greater than 20 g/d or suspicion of alcohol dependence
- Active substance abuse
- Liver cirrhosis
- History of dysmotility or delayed gastric emptying
- Pregnancy or breastfeeding
- History of eating disorder, or a serious or uncontrolled psychiatric illness that could compromise understanding or compliance with visits and device removal
- Patients unable or unwilling to take proton pump inhibitors for the duration of the device implant

Supplies needed for the placement of IGB
- Standard gastroscope
- Balloon system placement/fill catheter with guidewire
- Balloon connecting tube with 3-way valve and saline bag spine
- A 500- to 1000-mL bag of saline with methylene blue
- A 50-mL syringe

Medication for symptom management should be preordered for the patient, in order to be available to the patient immediately upon discharge. The patients and providers should not wait for symptoms to trigger the ordering of medication, because this may delay or decrease their overall tolerance after balloon placement. In our institution we provide patients with instruction for medication management before the procedure for balloon placement, and preorder the following medication regimen:

- Omeprazole, 40 mg, every 12 hours on empty stomach for the first 2 weeks, starting 2 weeks before implantation. After that, if the patient has no significant reflux symptoms they can switch to 20 mg once daily. The patients are instructed to continue this medication for the whole duration of device implantation (6 months). Some may experience an increase in gastroesophageal reflux disease symptoms after balloon removal, which may continue for 2 to 3 weeks.

- Metoclopramide,10 mg, 3 times a day before meals for the first week and then as needed.
- Scopolamine patch (1×) every 72 hours (after second patch, subsequent patches only if nauseated) for the first 1 to 2 weeks.
- Ondansetron 4 to 8 mg every 4 hours for the first 2 to 3 days and then as needed for nausea.
- Optional aprepitant for the first 3 days after balloon placement (120 mg, 80 mg, 80 mg). Usually not covered by insurance, and out-of-pocket cost need to be added to overall procedure cost for the patient.

In the immediate postprocedure period, patients should be given guidelines with dietary recommendations and restrictions. This particularly applies to the first 1 to 3 days, leading into the first 2 weeks after balloon placement. Typical recommendations mirror the following:

- *Day 1 to 2*: clear liquids only.
- *Day 3 to 14*: full liquid diet limited to 1000 to 1200 kcal/d. The first 2 weeks are a period of rapid weight loss for patients.
- *Day 15 to 21*: soft food, 1200 to 1500 kcal/d with 60 to 80 g of protein per day.
- *Thereafter*: normal textured foods. Patients are advised to maintain a healthy balanced diet. Weight loss continues, but at a slower pace.
- *Last 1 to 2 months*: Weight loss has usually plateaued at that point. Patients are instructed to observe and record their food intake to learn how much food they need to maintain their weight loss.
- *After balloon removal*: Patients continue with monthly dietician follow-up to ensure maintenance of weight loss.

Clear liquid diet phase
- Low-calorie, low acid fruit juices
- Weak coffee or tea
- Fat-free clear broth or soup
- Low-calorie/sugar-free gelatin
- Sugar-free popsicles (no fruit or cream)

Full liquid diet phase
- All foods included in clear liquid phase
- Low-fat yogurt drinks
- Skim milk/almond milk
- Thinned cream of wheat or oatmeal
- Protein shakes made with protein powders

Pureed/soft food phase progressing to normal textured foods
- Patients should stick to soft foods only, that is, foods that can be swallowed without significant chewing required
- Solids should be introduced gradually
- Cook all food, avoid raw food
- Limit bread, pasta, rice, and other because as they may stick to the balloon and cause halitosis
- Recommend ½ glass of water 30 minutes before and 30 minutes after eating to "rinse" the balloon

Patients require active monitoring in the postplacement period to evaluate for early symptoms and improve tolerance (**Table 2**). Dehydration can be prevented or treated early through use of intravenous fluids and electrolyte replacement.

Table 2
Common postprocedure issues and management

Issues	Management	Other Options
Postprocedure nausea and vomiting	Ondansetron 8 mg po tid × 3–5 d Metoclopramide 10 mg marijuana id × 3–5 d Scopolamine patch 1 mg/72 h × 6–9 d (precautions with glaucoma)	Prochorperazine (Compazine) 10 mg suppository Ondansetron sublingual tablet 4, 8 mg Aprepitant (Emend) 125 mg, 80 mg IV antinausea therapy in the office
Dehydration	Ensure adequate po intake in the first 2–3 d after placement by telephone interview IV fluids and antiemetics in the office	
Reflux symptoms	Proton pump inhibitor po daily × time of implantation + 2 wk before placement, or any other proton pump inhibitor	Increased doses/frequency
Concern for spontaneous deflation	Patient education Methylene blue 1–2 vials in balloon Abdominal radiograph	CT scan Endoscopy
Malodorous breath	Carbonated drinks × 2–3 d Liquid diet × 2–3 d	Probiotics
Vomiting after the first 2 wk	Review dietary indiscretions Clear liquid and full liquid diet for a few days Antiemetics	Consider endoscopy to rule out gastric ulceration if no response Imaging to rule out obstruction
Insufficient weight loss	Patient education Compliance with dietician's visits	Consider online/remote nutritional programs such as Orbera Health
Nutritional deficiencies	Consider hypokalemia, vitamin D, iron, folate, vitamin B_{12}, and thiamine deficiencies with rapid weight loss	

Abbreviations: CT, computed tomography; IV, intravenous; po, orally.

At the conclusion of 6 months, the balloon may be removed safely. Patients are asked to stay on a full liquid diet for 3 to 4 days before removal, a clear liquid diet for the preceding 24 to 36 hours, and to remain NPO for 12 hours before procedure. An upper endoscopy is then performed to confirm positioning of the balloon and exclude the presence of residual food. A needle instrument is then inserted through the endoscope to puncture the balloon within the stomach. The balloon content is aspirated through wall suction in the unit. The deflated balloon may then be grasped with a wire grasper and removed along with the endoscope. Follow-up endoscopy should be performed to ensure there is no injury to the esophagus or the stomach. We recommend that this procedure is done under general anesthesia, because solid food pieces may still be found in the stomach and there is an increased risk of aspiration. The patients continue their follow-up with a nutritionist or a life-style coach for another 6 months. A summary of our dietary and lifestyle instructions is presented in **Table 3**.

THE FUTURE OF INTRAGASTRIC BALLOONS

Several additional devices are being investigated, but have not yet been approved by the FDA for use in the United States.

The Elipse device is delivered in a capsule form that is swallowed, rather than placed endoscopically. This device is filled with up to 550 mL of normal saline via an attached catheter that, after filling, is released from the balloon. This device is unique in that it does not require endoscopy to remove it. At 4 months, a valve in the balloon is preset to open and deflate automatically. The Elipse is made of a thinner silicone material that is designed to pass uneventfully through the gastrointestinal tract.[27] In a recent prospective trial of 34 patients, there were no cases of intestinal obstruction, although

Table 3 Dietary and Lifestyle Instructions for patients	
General Nutritional and Lifestyle Advice	
Education about nutrition	Understanding energy balance. Reading food labels. Estimating portion size. Estimating calorie and sodium content.
Dietary instructions	Eat 3 meals a day and 2 small snacks. Eat slowly and chew food well. Aim to chew meat and chicken 20 times. Slowly sip water after meals. Avoid foods with high sugar content and limit alcohol to 1–2 glasses/wk. Drink eight 8-oz glasses of water a day. Avoid carbonated drinks in the first 4 wk. May sip Seltzer slowly afterward.
Lifestyle instructions	Avoid lying down shortly after eating and wait at least 2 h before going to bed. Some discomfort may occur lying down or lying on your side. You can change sides and/or use pillows to sit up Exercise and/or walk for 15–30 min or more daily. Avoid more than 2–3 alcoholic beverages per week
Long-term weight loss success tips	Eat high-protein breakfast regularly. Avoid foods with high sugar content, or food made of starch. Check your weight at least once a week. Exercise regularly, 3 times a week. In addition, walk every day for at least 1 hour. Buy a pedometer and aim for 10,000 steps a day. Avoid snacking between meals and eating late at night. Avoid processed snacks such as potato chips, tortilla chips, most granola bars. Many of these processed foods have ingredients with unclear benefits, may stimulate your appetite, and are usually high in sodium, fat, and starches.

4 balloons were vomited by the patients. Abdominal pain, nausea, vomiting, and early removal owing to intolerance were among the most common side effects. Total body weight loss was 10%.[21]

The Spatz balloon is an adjustable balloon system that may remain implanted for 12 months. The balloon has an attached catheter that can be used to increase or decrease the balloon volume. Thus, if the patient has reached a weight loss plateau, seen usually after the second month of balloon implantation, the balloon's volume can be increased during an additional endoscopy, or conversely, brought down in cases of intolerance.[28] An early trial of 18 patients showed a mean weight loss of 15.6 kg at 24 weeks and 24.4 kg at 52 weeks.[19] More than 10,000 Spatz balloons have been implanted worldwide, with information available on efficacy and adverse events.

Newer technologies are allowing the design and development of various other swallowable space-occupying devices. Devices with more durability and customizability are on the horizon, allowing gastroenterologists to have even more options for the treatment of obese patients.

Currently, the IGBs offer a safe and effective weight loss option for patients. Cost and access are an issue for many, but better insurance coverage in the future and decreased costs with nonendoscopic options will lead to wider availability of this promising treatment modality.

REFERENCES

1. Morino M, Toppino M, Forestieri P, et al. Mortality after bariatric surgery: analysis of 13,871 morbidly obese patients from a national registry. Ann Surg 2007;246: 1007–9.
2. Martin M, Beekley A, Kjorstad R, et al. Socioeconomic disparities in eligibility and access to bariatric surgery: a national population-based analysis. Surg Obes Relat Dis 2010;6:8–15.
3. World Health Organization. Obesity: preventing and managing the global epidemic. Geneva (Switzerland): Report of a WHO Consultation on Obesity; 1998.
4. Ulicny K, Goldberg SJ, Harper WJ, et al. Surgical complications of the Garren-Edwards Gastric Bubble. Surg Gynecol Obstet 1988;166(6):535–40.
5. Mathus-Vliegen E. Endoscopic treatment: the past, the present and the future. Best Pract Res Clin Gastroenterol 2014;28(4):685–702.
6. Obalon. 2016. [Online]. Available at: http://www.obalon.com/. Accessed September 17, 2016.
7. Gomez V. Baseline gastric emptying and its change in response to diverse endoscopic bariatric therapies predict weight change after intervention. Obesity 2016; 24(9):1849–53.
8. Mion F, Napoléon B, Roman S, et al. Effects of IOntragastric Balloon on Gastric Empyting and Plasma Ghrelin levels in Non morbid obese patients. Obes Surg 2005;15(4):510–6.
9. Apollo Endosurgery. Obera managed weight loss system. 2016. [Online]. Available at: www.obera.com. Accessed September 17, 2016.
10. ReShape non surgical weight loss procedure. ReShape Medical; 2016 [Online]. Available at: http://pro.reshapeready.com/about-reshape/. Accessed September 17, 2016.
11. Genco A, Bruni T, Doldi SB, et al. BioEnterics intragastric balloon: the Italian experience with 2,515 patients. Obes Surg 2005;15:1161–4.
12. Kotzampassi K. Intragastric balloon as an alternative restrictive procedure for morbid obesity. Ann Gastroenterol 2005;19(3):285–8.

13. Imaz I, Martínez-Cervell C, García-Alvarez EE, et al. Safety and Effectiveness of the Intragastric Balloon for obesity. A meta-analysis. Obes Surg 2008;18:841–6.
14. Ponce J, Woodman G, Swain J, et al. The REDUCE pivotal trial: a prospective randomized controlled pivotal trial of a dual intragastric balloon for the treatment of obesity. Surg Obes Relat Dis 2015;11(4):874–81.
15. Martinez-Brocca M, Belda O, Parejo J, et al. Intragastric balloon-induced satiety in not mediated by modification in fasting or postprandial plasma ghrelin levels in morbid obesity. Obes Surg 2007;17:649–57.
16. Lee YM, Low HC, Lim LG, et al. Intragastric balloon significantly improves nonalcoholic fatty liver disease activity score in obese patients with nonalcoholic hepatohepatitis: a pilot study. Gastrointest Endosc 2012;76(4):756–60.
17. Farina MG, Baratta R, Nigro A, et al. Intragastric balloon in association with lifestyle and/or pharmacotherapy in the long-term management of obesity. Obes Surg 2012;22:565–71.
18. Mathus-Vliegen E. Gastro-oesophageal reflux in obese subject: influence of overweight weight loss and chronic gastric balloon distension. Scand J Gastroenterol 2002;11:1246–52.
19. Machytka E, Klvana P, Kornbluth A, et al. Adjustable intragastric balloons: a 12-month pilot trial in endoscopic weight loss management. Obes Surg 2011;21(10):1499–507.
20. Chuttani R. Abstract ET012. Presented at SAGES Annual Meeting, Boston, March 16-19, 2016.
21. Cuttani RI. Digestive Disease Week, San Diego, May 20–25, 2016.
22. Sullivan S, Swain D. The Obalon swallowable 6-month balloon system is more effective than moderate intensity lifestyle therapy alone: results from a 6-month randomized sham controlled trial. Gastroenterology 2016;150(4)(Suppl 1):S1267.
23. Fuller N, Pearson S, Lau NS, et al. An intragastric balloon in the treatment of obese individuals with metabolic syndrome: a randomized controlled study. Obesity 2013;21:1561–70.
24. Popov V, Ou A, Schulman A, et al. The impact of intragastric balloons on obesity-related co-morbidities: a systematic review and meta-analysis. Gastroenterology 2016;150(4)(Suppl 1):S85.
25. Popov V, Thompson CC, Kumar N, et al. Effect of intragastric balloons on liver enzymes: a systematic review and meta-analysis. Dig Dis Sci 2016;61(9):2477–87.
26. Abu Dayyeh BK, Kumar N, Edmundowicz SA, et al. ASGE bariatric endoscopy task force systemic review and meta-analysis assessing the ASGE PIVI thresholds for adopting endoscopic bariatric therapies. Gastrointest Endosc 2015; 82(3):425–38.e5.
27. Allurion. 2016. [Online]. Available at: http://allurion.com/the-elipse-gastric-balloon/. Accessed September 17, 2016.
28. Spatz Medical. 2016. [Online]. Available at: http://www.spatzmedical.com/advantages.html. Accessed September 17, 2016.
29. Brooks J, Srivastava ED, Mathus-Vliegen EM. One-year adjustable intragastric balloons: results in 73 consecutive patients in the U.K. Obes Surg 2014;24(5):813–9.

Gastric Plication

Nitin Kumar, MD

KEYWORDS

- Endoscopic sleeve gastroplasty • Primary obesity surgery endolumenal
- Articulating Endoscopic Circular stapler

KEY POINTS

- Gastric plication, like all endoscopic bariatric therapies, should be delivered in the context of a multidisciplinary weight management program.
- Endoscopic sleeve gastroplasty has demonstrated efficacy and is entering clinical practice.
- Primary obesity surgery endolumenal has shown efficacy and is under review by the US Food and Drug Administration.
- The Articulating Endoscopic Circular (ACE) stapler and TransOral Gastroplasty system (TOGa) can also be used to perform gastric plication, although commercial status is uncertain.
- As with medical or surgical weight loss techniques, it is important to continue long-term clinical weight management to maintain weight loss.

INTRODUCTION

More than 81 million Americans have obesity, and more Americans are overweight.[1] Diet and lifestyle management programs are limited in effectiveness by physiologic responses, and despite their wide availability, the prevalence of obesity has grown markedly in recent decades.[2] Medications that show moderate efficacy have recently been approved by the US Food and Drug Administration (FDA). Effective therapies, such as bariatric surgery, have not been used broadly because of concerns about invasiveness and limited access because of coverage restrictions.[3]

Endoscopic therapies for obesity can fill the efficacy, invasiveness, and availability gap between conservative measures and bariatric surgery. Various endoscopic bariatric therapies act on the stomach, small intestine, or both. Their mechanisms of action may be analogous to bariatric surgeries, for example, gastric restriction or intestinal bypass. Others, such as aspiration therapy, use mechanisms not seen in bariatric surgery. One restrictive technique is gastric plication. One current endoscopic technique for gastric plication is endoscopic sleeve gastroplasty (ESG). In its

Disclosure Statement: The author is a consultant for Obalon.
Bariatric Endoscopy Institute, 1450 W Lake Street, Suite 101, Addison, IL 60101, USA
E-mail address: nkumar@obesityendoscopy.org

contemporary form, this procedure uses endoscopic suturing to remodel all or part of the stomach into a tubular sleeve, reducing both gastric volume and accommodation ability and perhaps affecting gastric motility (**Fig. 1**). Other techniques have also been studied. Two techniques use staplers—transoral gastroplasty (TOGa; Satiety Inc, Palo Alto, CA) and the Articulating Endoscopic Circular (ACE; Boston Scientific Corporation, Natick, MA) stapler. Another, under review by the FDA, uses the Incisionless Operating Platform (IOP; USGI Medical, San Clemente, CA) to perform the primary obesity surgery endolumenal (POSE).

ENDOLUMINAL VERTICAL GASTROPLASTY

Endoscopic suturing has evolved over time. The first endoscopic treatment of obesity using endoscopic suturing was for revision of Roux-en-Y gastric bypass, using the Bard EndoCinch (Davol, Murray Hill, NJ), a suction-based suturing device originally intended for endoscopic treatment of gastroesophageal reflux disease.[4,5] The Endo-Cinch was then applied for the primary treatment of obesity, by performing endoluminal vertical gastroplasty, an analogue of a bariatric surgery called *vertical banded gastroplasty*.[6]

ENDOSCOPIC SLEEVE GASTROPLASTY
Superficial Thickness Suturing

A subsequent iteration of the EndoCinch, the RESTORe endoscopic suturing device (Davol) was used to perform the first endoscopic sleeve gastroplasty. RESTORe could perform deeper-thickness suturing than the EndoCinch and did not need to be removed and reinserted for suture reloading. ESG was performed in the TRIM trial, with placement of an average of 6 plications to approximate the anterior and posterior walls of the stomach. The prospective TRIM trial performed at 2 centers included 18 subjects.[7] The subjects lost 27.7% $\pm$ 21.9% of their excess weight (11.0 $\pm$ 10 kg). Waist circumference decreased by 12.6 $\pm$ 9.5 cm. However, endoscopic follow-up found that suture placement was not durable.

Full-Thickness Suturing

The OverStitch (Apollo Endosurgery, Austin, TX) has made full-thickness endoscopic suturing possible. The device can rapidly place full-thickness sutures in several configurations, including interrupted and running stitches. It can be reloaded without removal and reinsertion. The device has an actuating handle, which attaches to the endoscope handle, and a needle driver, which attaches to the endoscope tip. At

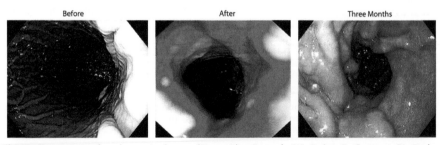

Before   After   Three Months

Fig. 1. Formation of endoscopic sleeve. (*From* Abu Dayyeh BK, Rajan E, Gostout CJ. Endoscopic sleeve gastroplasty: a potential endoscopic alternative to surgical sleeve gastrectomy for treatment of obesity. Gastrointest Endosc 2013;78(3):534; with permission.)

this time, a double channel endoscope is required. One channel is used for a suture anchor catheter, and the other can be used for a tissue helix. The helix is a catheter with a retractable corkscrew tip, which can be used to securely grasp tissue and bring it into the working area of the OverStitch. After the stitches have been placed, the suture is tightened and secured with a combined suture-cutting catheter and cinch tag placement device. The device has been approved by the FDA for tissue apposition and has been used for a variety of gastrointestinal procedures.[8] A comparison of full-thickness suturing with superficial thickness suturing showed greater efficacy (weight loss after gastric bypass revision) using the same technique, suggesting that full-thickness suturing may be associated with greater durability.[9]

A standardized full-thickness ESG technique was developed in an international multicenter fashion starting in April 2012.[10,11] Multiple iterations of the procedure were evaluated for feasibility, safety, and efficacy at centers in India, Panama, and the Dominican Republic, followed by the United States and Spain. Obese patients who did not respond to diet and lifestyle modification were included, and patients with prior gastric surgery, eating disorders, bleeding disorders, psychiatric disease, and gastrointestinal disease were excluded.

Procedure Development

The initial 5 human cases in India evaluated the safety and feasibility of several stitch patterns to optimize efficiency.[10] Argon plasma coagulation was used to create dotted lines from the gastroesophageal junction to the antrum in a longitudinal fashion—one along the anterior wall and one along the posterior wall, toward the greater curvature side of the midline. Running stitches were created in a triangular fashion, including 6 to 12 tissue acquisitions each. The suturing was started in the fundus, which required working in retroflexion. After each stitch, the endoscope was rotated and moved distally to start the next stitch. The lumen toward the greater curvature was excluded. The tissue helix was used for tissue acquisition in some stitches, but suction was used to bring tissue into the device in others. Because of the challenge of working in retroflexion and use of suction to acquire tissue, procedure time was 3.5 ± 0.5 hours. There was no free intraperitoneal air on chest radiograph, and there were no reported significant adverse events during the procedure or during the follow-up period.

The second phase of procedure development started with the final technique refined in the first stage, and assessed time efficiency in 22 patients. The longitudinal argon plasma coagulation lines were eliminated because they did not remain in a consistent position after suturing began. Because free air had not been seen on chest x-ray during the first phase, the tissue helix was used for each stitch placement to ensure full-thickness stitches. The suturing was initiated in the antrum and moved proximally to the fundus, which eliminated the need for cumbersome retroflexed suturing for much of the procedure. Additionally, this allowed the fundus to be pulled downward. Rather than using up to 12 stitches per suture, 6 stitches were used (at most) before securing the stitches. This action reduced complexity, and the risk of stitch release from tissue caused by high suture tension. During the second phase, it was noted that full-thickness suture placement resulted in free air on chest radiograph; insufflation was modified to use carbon dioxide. A subset of patients was operated on using only interrupted stitches, which resulted in durable stitch placement but was time consuming. However, this technique was incorporated to add to sleeve durability, and a row of interrupted stitches was placed medially to the suture line after the sleeve was created.

The third phase was performed in the Dominican Republic, the United States, and Spain to assess the efficacy of the final technique in 77 patients with a body mass index

(BMI) of 36.1 ± 0.6 kg/m^2. Nausea and epigastric pain were routinely reported, as well as transient epigastric pain, in the postoperative period. No significant adverse events were reported to the prospective registry. Patients at some centers were admitted for 24 hours after the procedure, whereas others were discharged home on the same day. Preliminary data showed weight loss of 17.9 ± 1.3 kg, or 17.4 ± 1.1% total weight loss (TWL), at 12 months.

Procedure Technique

At most centers, ESG is currently performed using the standardized technique created in the procedure development process. General anesthesia with endotracheal intubation is necessary. An esophageal overtube should be used to protect the oropharynx and esophagus. The use of a cephalosporin antibiotic for prophylaxis is advisable. The patient should be placed in a partial left lateral/supine position. Because of long procedure times, intraoperative venous thromboembolism prophylaxis should be considered. Preoperative and postoperative antiemetics can reduce nausea. In its current and most broadly applied form, full-thickness ESG is performed by placing a series of running stitches, each made of 6 stitch placements in a 2-triangle configuration. A triangular stitch is placed from the anterior gastric wall to the greater curvature to the posterior gastric wall, and a second triangle is placed before the suture is cinched and secured. These stitches are placed in a series, beginning in the antrum, and moving proximally to the fundus. This stitch pattern excludes the gastric lumen along the greater curvature and shortens the stomach, resulting in the creation of a tubular sleeve along the lesser curvature. The suture line along the lateral sleeve is reinforced with multiple interrupted stitches. Routine use of the helix is recommended to aid full-thickness stitch placement and to avoid injury to structures adjacent to the stomach. The procedure entails long operating times and requires familiarity with torquing the endoscope, avoidance of crossed sutures in the setting of multiple running stitch placements, and management of suture tension to avoid suture pull-through.

Clinical Results

Over time, published series show the safety and efficacy of ESG.

- A series of 10 patients with mean BMI of 45.2 kg/m^2 reported 6-month TWL of 33.0 kg, equivalent to 30% excess weight loss (EWL).[12] There was a significant improvement in postprandial glucose, with a 36% decrease in area under the curve.
- A prospective study of 25 subjects with average BMI of 38.5 ± 4.6 kg/m^2 reported TWL of 18.7 ± 10.7% after 12 months.[13] In the setting of multidisciplinary follow-up, the number of visits to a nutritionist and psychologist was a predictor of superior weight loss results, underscoring the importance of clinical follow-up after the procedure. In one case, the procedure was endoscopically revised to restore gastric plication.
- An international multicenter series including 126 patients with average BMI of 36.2 kg/m^2 reported BMI decrease to 29.8 ± 1.4 kg/m^2 after 12 months.[11] Weight decreased from 101.6 ± 2.3 kg to 81.8 ± 3.8 kg/m^2 after 12 months. No serious adverse events were reported.
- A prospective study including 25 subjects with average BMI of 35.5 kg/m^2 reported 3 serious adverse events: perigastric inflammatory serous fluid collection, pulmonary embolism, and pneumoperitoneum with pneumothorax.[14] At 12 months, EWL was 54 ± 40% (n = 10) and 45 ± 41% at 20 months (n = 8). A detailed analysis of motility and neurohormonal changes was performed in

4 patients: after 3 months, ESG decreased the caloric intake required to achieve maximum satiety by 59%, meal duration decreased from 35.2 ± 9.9 minutes to 11.5 ± 2.3 minutes, and fasting and postprandial ghrelin levels decreased by 29.4%. Insulin sensitivity also increased significantly.

- A multicenter series of 242 patients (including patients reported in other series) reported 19.8% TWL after 18 months.[15] There was a serious adverse event rate of 2%, with report of a perigastric fluid collection treated with percutaneous drainage and antibiotics, self-limited hemorrhage from splenic laceration, pulmonary embolism, and pneumoperitoneum/pneumothorax.
- ESG has been endoscopically revised to address a plateau in weight loss.[16] A case report described a 60-year-old woman with baseline BMI of 33.5 kg/m^2 who reached BMI of 26.5 kg/m^2 and 21% TWL 1 year after ESG. However, her weight loss subsided. She had an endoscopy, which showed prior gastroplasty with loosened sutures. Two layers of running stitches were placed to approximate opposing gastric walls. A gentamicin lavage was performed to prevent infection, and she was discharged home on the same day. One month later, she had an additional 8% TWL, reaching BMI of 24.4% and 27% TWL.
- Other adverse events have been reported, including a case report describing onset of abdominal pain and vomiting 12 days after ESG.[17] Computed tomography scan showed a 3.3 × 2.9 × 3.7 cm fundic fluid collection along the greater curvature, consistent with a perigastric collection. The patient was given antibiotics—a dose of intravenous ertapenem followed by oral ciprofloxacin, 500 mg twice daily, and metronidazole, 400 mg 3 times daily for 7 days. The collection resolved on follow-up imaging.

Mechanism

ESG (and the preceding vertical gastroplasty) are often analogized to surgical sleeve gastrectomy. However, ESG differs in important ways. Whereas sleeve gastrectomy permanently alters the stomach with excision of gastric tissue, ESG remodels its shape. ESG is less invasive, but sleeve gastrectomy excises ghrelin-producing tissue. Whereas sleeve gastrectomy is permanent, ESG may be reversible, and its durability is being studied. Therefore, ESG is not necessarily an analogue of sleeve gastrectomy. This fact was underscored when the mechanism of ESG was studied by Abu Dayyeh and colleagues.[12] ESG seems to slow gastric emptying, whereas sleeve gastrectomy speeds it. Further investigation of the mechanism, neurohormonal effects, and subsequent change in comorbidities is ongoing. There is potential for ESG to be combined with endoscopic small bowel interventions, medications, or other technologies with complimentary mechanisms to potentiate the effect of ESG.

OTHER GASTRIC RESTRICTIVE PROCEDURES
Primary Obesity Surgery Endolumenal

POSE creates gastric restriction using the Incisionless Operating Platform device (IOP). IOP comprises a 4-channel platform, with a tissue helix, tissue grasper and suture cutter, suture anchor catheter, and a channel for a 4.9-mm endoscope for visualization. The IOP can create plications in the stomach by apposing tissue, deploying a full-thickness stitch, and then anchoring it in place. The POSE procedure starts with IOP in retroflexion, and placement of 2 parallel lines of 4 to 5 plications (**Fig. 2**). Once the fundic apex has been reduced to the level of the gastroesophageal junction, the IOP is restored to the forward view. Another 3 to 4 plications are placed at the distal gastric body across from the incisura.

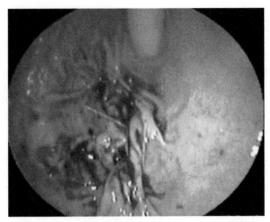

Fig. 2. Fundic plications in POSE. (*From* Espinós JC, Turró R, Moragas G, et al. Gastrointestinal Physiologic Changes and Their Relationship to Weight Loss Following the POSE Procedure. Obes Surg 2016;26(5):1083; with permission.)

One study including 45 subjects with mean BMI of 36.7 ± 3.8 kg/m^2 reported TWL of 15.5 ± 6.1% after 6 months, with BMI decrease of 5.8 kg/m^2.[18] There was 1 report of chest pain and 1 report of low-grade fever. Another study including 147 subjects with pre-POSE BMI of 38.0 ± 4.8 kg/m^2 found 15.1 ± 7.8% TWL at 1 year; no significant adverse events were reported.[19] The randomized sham-controlled ESSENTIAL trial included 332 subjects with average BMI of 36.0 ± 2.4 kg/m^2, with 221 assigned to POSE and 111 to sham.[20] Preliminary data report that mean TWL in the POSE group was 3.6 times the weight loss in the sham arm at 12 months, and responders (those with >5% TWL) achieved 11.5% TWL at 1 year. Procedure-related adverse events were reported in 11 POSE subjects and 1 sham subject, with all presenting within the first week. The IOP is under review for POSE by the FDA.

Transoral Gastroplasty

Transoral gastroplasty was performed using a procedure-specific endoscopic stapler (TOGa). An endoscope is inserted through the device and then retroflexed for visualization. The esophagus must be dilated to 60F with a Savary-Gilliard (R) Dilator (Cook Medical, Bloomington, IN) to accommodate the device, which is inserted over a guidewire.[21] The TOGa uses a vacuum to appose the gastric walls, and then a stapler secures a 4.5-cm sleeve with titanium staples. After the device is removed and reloaded, it is fired again to create an 8-cm-long sleeve (2 cm in diameter) along the lesser curvature of the stomach. A study (using the first-generation device) including 21 subjects with average BMI of 43.3 kg/m^2 reported transient pain, dysphagia, nausea, and vomiting as adverse events.[22] Weight loss at 6 months averaged 12 kg, equivalent to 24.4% EWL. A multicenter study of 67 subjects reported adverse events including an instance of asymptomatic pneumoperitoneum and another of respiratory insufficiency.[23] After 12 months, the BMI ≥40 group experienced 52.2% EWL and the BMI less than 40 group achieved 41.3% EWL. Additionally, hemoglobin A1c levels declined from 7.0% to 5.7%, and there was improvement in high-density lipoprotein and triglyceride levels. The device has not been commercialized.

Articulating Endoscopic Circular Stapler

The ACE endoscopic stapler has a rotating, retroflexing head. The device is 16 mm in diameter and accommodates a 5-mm endoscope for visualization. Tissue is acquired

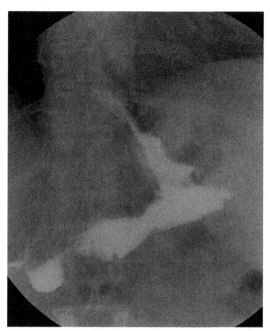

Fig. 3. Contrast radiograph after ACE stapler plication. (*From* Verlaan T, Paulus GF, Mathus-Vliegen EM, et al. Endoscopic gastric volume reduction with a novel articulating plication device is safe and effective in the treatment of obesity (with video). Gastrointest Endosc 2015;81(2):316; with permission.)

with vacuum suction, and then the stapler deploys 10 mm plastic ring with and 8 full-thickness titanium staples. Gastric volume reduction can be performed by creating 8 fundic plications and 2 antral plications (**Fig. 3**). A study including 17 subjects with median BMI of 40.2 kg/m^2 reported a median procedure time of 123 minutes.[24] Adverse events included transient abdominal pain in 7 subjects and transient sore throat, nausea, vomiting, constipation, and diarrhea. Medial weight loss was 34.9% EWL (interquartile range, 17.8–46.6). Some patients (11 of 17) had follow-up endoscopy at 12 months, which found 6 to 9 extant plications in each subject, with persistence of gastric volume reduction.

SUMMARY

Endoscopic gastric plication techniques have proven effective for weight loss. These procedures offer the potential for higher efficacy than conservative modalities, such as medications and lifestyle modifications, and lower invasiveness than bariatric surgery. At this time, POSE is under review by the FDA, and endoscopic sleeve gastroplasty is gaining acceptance. Although ESG is technically demanding and has been associated with long procedure times in its current form, the procedure continues to be refined. In the meantime, expertise in endoscopic suturing is crucial before applying the technique. Although long-term durability remains to be determined, if needed, ESG can be repeated to reconstruct the sleeve. Gastric plication procedures, as with any endoscopic bariatric therapy, should be applied in the setting of a multidisciplinary weight management program with long-term follow-up.

REFERENCES

1. Ward ZJ, Long MW, Resch SC, et al. Redrawing the US obesity landscape: bias-corrected estimates of state-specific adult obesity prevalence. PLoS One 2016; 11(3):e0150735.
2. Ochner CN, Barrios DM, Lee CD, et al. Biological mechanisms that promote weight regain following weight loss in obese humans. Physiol Behav 2013;0: 106–13.
3. Nguyen NT, Vu S, Kim E, et al. Trends in utilization of bariatric surgery, 2009-2012. Surg Endosc 2015;30(7):2723–7.
4. Thompson CC, Carr-Locke DL, Saltzman J. Peroral endoscopic repair of staple-line dehiscence in Roux-en-Y gastric bypass: a less invasive approach. Gastroenterology 2004;126(Suppl 2)A.
5. Thompson, CC. Endoscopic gastric bypass defect repair. U.S. Patent 8,623,009, Filed. April 5, 2006. Published Jan 7, 2014.
6. Fogel R, De Fogel J, Bonilla Y, et al. Clinical experience of transoral suturing for an endoluminal vertical gastroplasty: 1-year follow-up in 64 patients. Gastrointest Endosc 2008;68(1):51–8.
7. Brethauer SA, Chand B, Schauer PR, et al. Transoral gastric volume reduction for weight management: technique and feasibility in 18 patients. Surg Obes Relat Dis 2010;6(6):689–94.
8. Abu Dayyeh BK, Acosta A, Camilleri M, et al. Endoscopic sleeve gastroplasty alters gastric physiology and induces loss of body weight in obese individuals. Clin Gastroenterol Hepatol 2017;15(1):37–43.
9. Kumar N, Thompson CC. Comparison of a superficial suturing device with a full-thickness suturing device for transoral outlet reduction (with videos). Gastrointest Endosc 2014;79(6):984–9.
10. Kumar N, Sahdala HN, Shaikh S, et al. Endoscopic sleeve gastroplasty for primary therapy of obesity: Initial human cases. Gastroenterology 2014;146(5): S571–2.
11. Kumar N, Lopez-Nava G, Sahdala HN, et al. Endoscopic sleeve gastroplasty: multicenter weight loss results. Gastroenterology 2015;148(4):S179.
12. Abu Dayyeh BK, Acosta A, Camilleri M, et al. Endoscopic sleeve gastroplasty alters gastric physiology and induces loss of body weight in obese individuals. Clin Gastroenterol Hepatol 2017;15(1):37–43.e1.
13. Sharaiha RZ, Kedia P, Kumta N, et al. Initial experience with endoscopic sleeve gastroplasty: technical success and reproducibility in the bariatric population. Endoscopy 2015;47(2):164–6.
14. Lopez-Nava G, Galvao M, Bautista-Castaño I, et al. Endoscopic sleeve gastroplasty with 1-year follow-up: factors predictive of success. Endosc Int Open 2016;4:E222–7.
15. Lopez-Nava G, Sharaiha RZ, Neto MG, et al. Endoscopic sleeve gastroplasty for obesity: a multicenter study of 242 patients with 18 months follow-up. Gastroenterology 2016;150(4):S26.
16. Sharaiha RZ, Kedia P, Kumta N, et al. Endoscopic sleeve plication for revision of sleeve gastrectomy. Gastrointest Endosc 2015;81(4):1004.
17. Barola S, Agnihotri A, Khashab MA, et al. Perigastric fluid collection after endoscopic sleeve gastroplasty. Endoscopy 2016;48(S 01):E340–1.
18. Espinós JC, Turró R, Mata A, et al. Early experience with the Incisionless Operating Platform™ (IOP) for the treatment of obesity: the Primary Obesity Surgery Endolumenal (POSE) procedure. Obes Surg 2013;23:1375–83.

19. López-Nava G, Bautista-Castaño I, Jimenez A, et al. The Primary Obesity Surgery Endolumenal (POSE) procedure: one-year patient weight loss and safety outcomes. Surg Obes Relat Dis 2015;11:861–5.
20. Sullivan S, Swain JM, Woodman G, et al. 12 month randomized sham controlled trial evaluating the safety and efficacy of targeted use of endoscopic suture anchors for primary obesity: The ESSENTIAL Study. Gastroenterology 2016;150(4 Suppl 1):S25–6.
21. Familiari P, Costamagna G, Bléro D, et al. Transoral gastroplasty for morbid obesity: a multicenter trial with a 1-year outcome. Gastrointest Endosc 2011;74: 1248–58.
22. Devière J, Ojeda Valdes G, Cuevas Herrera L, et al. Safety, feasibility and weight loss after transoral gastroplasty: First human multicenter study. Surg Endosc 2008;22:589–98.
23. Nanni G, Familiari P, Mor A, et al. Effectiveness of the Transoral Endoscopic Vertical Gastroplasty (TOGa): a good balance between weight loss and complications, if compared with gastric bypass and biliopancreatic diversion. Obes Surg 2012;22:1897–902.
24. Verlaan T, Paulus GF, Mathus-Vliegen EM, et al. Endoscopic gastric volume reduction with a novel articulating plication device is safe and effective in the treatment of obesity (with video). Gastrointest Endosc 2015;81:312–20.

he proximal duodenum. The tether traverses the pylorus, and the larger spherical b remains positioned in the antrum. The larger bulb intermittently engages the py- us during peristalsis, leading to transient gastric outlet obstruction, but then falls ck into the stomach, allowing for gastric content to pass through the pylorus inter- tently, hence the "shuttle" effect. In the clinical trials to date, the device placement r 6 to 12 months, followed by mandatory removal. Retrieval of the device requires use of a modified standard esophageal overtube using rat-tooth graspers and a re to unlock and uncoil the components of the proximal bulb, removing them ough the overtube and then grasping the outer skin and removing it from the mach.

he TPS has several key mechanisms of action that promote weight loss. The large b, although not sized as much as the water- or gas-filled balloons, represents a ce-occupying device, similar to IGBs, which partially reduces functional gastric ume. During antral contractions, the large bulb repeatedly engages the pylorus, sing intermittent obstruction. This action delays gastric emptying, prolongs gastric ommodation, and increases satiety. It is possible that the distal bulb is interacting duodenal mucosa and incretin signaling, although this remains to be elucidated.

2014, a prospective, nonrandomized single-center clinical trial reported the feasi- y, safety, and efficacy of the TPS device.[14] A total of 20 patients were enrolled, all hich had a BMI between 30 and 50 kg/m^2. Proton pump inhibitors were adminis- d for all patients during the length of the study. The device was safely deployed removed in all 20 patients. At 3- and 6-month follow-up, 25.1% and 44.0% excess ght loss (EWL) were observed, respectively. Ninety percent of study patients aled maximum weight loss at the time of device removal, which suggested the sibility of longer-term weight loss potential. Two patients required early device oval due to gastric ulceration.

ollowing strong pilot data, the pivotal ENDObesity II study was initiated in the ed States, which represents a multicenter, randomized, sham-controlled clinical The target study population (n = 270, 2:1 randomization for the device) includes ents who have failed lifestyle changes or medical therapy, with a BMI of 30.0 to . The study has completed subject enrollment, with early observation being highly uraging for safely producing weight loss.

e TPS device is designed for temporary placement and does not fundamentally the gastrointestinal anatomy. Similar to IGBs, the indications for TPS placement be both for primary obesity management and as a bridge to bariatric surgery. This ce may also prove to be useful for the pediatric population. In addition to defining eight loss potential, translational research studies investigating the correspond- eurohormonal signaling are warranted to better characterize the antiobesity e of the TPS device.

es/Techniques Affecting Gastric Wall or Postbypass Stomal Compliance

scopic sclerotherapy

refaced in the article dedicated to endoscopic revision of Roux-en-Y ss (RYGB), weight regain after bariatric surgery is a common complica d anatomic defects can contribute to weight regain, including gastric-g and dilated gastrojejunal (GJ) anastomosis. GJ aperture reduction n to curb weight regain and promote weight loss by potentially dela ying and increasing satiety.[15] option to alter compliance of the postbypass stoma and thereby y altering the kinetics of emptying may be accomplished with th ic sclerotherapy. Endoscopic sclerotherapy involves the injection

---

Selected Endoscopic Gastric Devices for Obesity

 CrossMark

Kartik Sampath, MD*, Richard I. Rothstein, MD

KEYWORDS

- Obesity • Stomach • Bariatric endoscopy • Therapeutic endoscopy • Devices

KEY POINTS

- Endoscopic devices can treat obesity and its related metabolic conditions by targeting key gastric anatomic and physiologic mechanisms.
- Recognizing the effect of the bariatric surgical interventions on gastric anatomy and physiology will contribute to the development of minimally invasive devices that can mimic these effects.
- There are many bariatric endoscopic devices, in various stages of development, targeting the stomach to promote caloric restriction and early satiety through anatomic and physiologic effects.
- The Transpyloric Shuttle involves several mechanisms of action, including occupying space, blocking the gastric exit, delaying gastric emptying, and potentially altering hormonal signaling.
- Gastric sclerotherapy, Botulinum toxin A injection, and radiofrequency ablation likely change gastric or postoperative stomal compliance or motility and emptying physiology and have been shown to produce weight loss. The ACE stapler represents a novel gastric volume-reducing device; further clinical study is needed.
- The Gelesis100 device and the Magnetic Weight Loss Capsule represent applications of material science and mechanical engineering, and with further study, can open avenues of clinical application.
- Randomized, blinded controlled trials are needed to determine the true effect of these unique devices beyond sham.

Financial Disclosures: Dr R.I. Rothstein has received research grant support from BaroNova (NCT02518685) and Barrx/Medtronic (NCT01910688) as well as consulting fees from Boston Scientific. He is on the scientific advisory board of Allurion.

Section of Gastroenterology and Hepatology, Department of Medicine, Dartmouth-Hitchcock Medical Center, Geisel School of Medicine at Dartmouth, One Medical Center Drive, Lebanon, NH 03756, USA
* Corresponding author.
E-mail address: kartik.sampath@hitchcock.org

SELECTED STOMACH TARGET DEVICES
Introduction

The obesity epidemic refers to the rising incidence of obesity worldwide and its impact on global health.[1] Bariatric surgery remains the most effective therapeutic option for obesity. At present, the overwhelming demand far exceeds the health care infrastructure capable of providing bariatric surgical services. Endoscopic therapy for obesity represents a potentially cost-effective, accessible, minimally invasive alternative that can function as both a primary therapeutic intervention and a bridge to bariatric surgery.

Endoscopic devices that target the stomach directly alter gastric physiology and promote weight loss by altering functional gastric volume, gastric emptying, gastric wall compliance, neurohormonal signaling, and satiety. Intragastric balloons (IGBs) and the endoscopic sleeve gastroplasty (ESG) procedure restrict functional gastric volume, which causes decreased caloric intake, increased satiety, and eventual weight loss. Aspiration therapy (AT) removes excess caloric ingestion directly from the stomach via an aspiration tube upon initial food bolus ingestion. These devices, in particular, are discussed extensively in separate respective articles. This article focuses on the non-IGB, non-ESG, non-AT stomach target devices that are currently in various stages of development and offer promise for future weight loss therapies.

It is important to understand the basic gastric physiology and motility, and the physiologic alterations of the bariatric surgical procedures, when evaluating the role and utility of current and future bariatric devices that target the stomach. With food ingestion, gastric accommodation initially produces fundic and corpus relaxation, with concurrent pyloric contraction and closure. The result is food bolus accumulation in the stomach. The mixing stage represents vagal nerve–mediated gastric antral contractions, which churn the food bolus against a contracted pylorus, with trituration of the ingesta. The emptying phase refers to pyloric relaxation with continued antral pump contraction. The food bolus then passes into the duodenum for further digestion and absorption. Neurohormonal signaling plays an instrumental role during the entire gastric digestive process. The integrated signaling that occurs with the act of eating, and through the process of gastric accommodation and emptying, has a complex interplay for the sensation of satiety and hunger and regulates processes that relate to energy balance, obesity, and related metabolic disorders. Understanding how medical and surgical bariatric interventions affect these mechanisms can direct the development of effective endoscopic devices. These devices may target anatomic processes and result in restriction of caloric intake or produce mal-digestion. It is likely that devices that will be most effective and durable will be ones that alter physiologic mechanisms, and much study is still needed to identify the changes that these devices may produce and which ones will be efficacious and safe. With other contributions detailing what is known about the currently approved gastric devices and techniques, and additional ones highlighting emerging new therapies, the authors focus on the remaining devices or techniques not covered elsewhere in this issue.

Devices/Techniques Affecting Gastric Emptying

Gastric botulinum toxin A injection

Botulinum toxin A (BTA) is an acetylcholinesterase inhibitor that functions as a long-acting inhibitor of both voluntary and smooth muscle contraction leading to a reversible paralytic-type effect. Direct injection into the gastric antral smooth muscle offers the potential to delay gastric emptying by moderating the propulsive contraction effect of the antral pump. In theory, pump inhibition leads to impaired gastric

emptying, increased satiety, inhibition of ghrelin release, decrea[s] eventual weight loss.

Preclinical animal studies were initially performed in rats. In 2000, parallel, randomized controlled study was performed whereby ra[t] laparotomy with gastric BTA injection, sham laparotomy, or contro[l] rotomy.[2] At 10-week follow-up, there was significant weight loss in t[he] the sham group (14.0% vs 4.4% [maximum weight loss as a per[cent] 2005, a follow-up randomized, sham-controlled study in a specific reiterated findings of significant weight loss in the BTA injection g[roup]

Numerous human pilot studies were subsequently performed. observational study demonstrated feasibility and safety of the method.[4] During a standard upper endoscopy, BTA was dire[cted] antral mucosa. Compared with baseline patient weights, the mean weight reduction at 1 month after BTA (121.8 kg vs 124. pilot studies investigated optimal BTA dosing administrations, gastric emptying; however, the results were generally equivoca[l]

In 2007, a randomized, sham-controlled study with 6-mont[h] weight reduction that was not statistically significant in the BTA a randomized controlled trial, performed in 2012, adminis[tered] throughout the stomach including the fundus.[8] The results not[ed signifi] cant weight loss at the interval 12-week follow-up.

In 2007, a randomized, sham-controlled trial revealed signifi[cant] vs 5.7 kg, P<.001) and body mass index (BMI) reduction P<.001) in the BTA group during 12-week follow-up.[9] This stud[y] also demonstrating significantly decreased gastric-emptying t[ime] (+18.9 vs −2.2, P<.05).

Given the equivocal data regarding mucosal-based gastric studies investigated submucosal BTA injection into the muscular[is] lot study was performed via endoscopic ultrasound–guided BTA [into] submucosa. At 16-week follow-up, the average body weight los[s] follow-up double-blinded, randomized, sham-controlled trial wa[s] At 24-week follow-up, there was no significant weight loss; delayed gastric emptying was observed in the 300-unit BTA inje[ction]

A 2015 meta-analysis was performed summarizing the 8 date, 5 of which were randomized controlled trials. The result[s] significant weight loss effects with gastric BTA treatment.[1] reviewing the study raised concerns regarding the study me[thods] the inclusion of non-randomized controlled trials in statistical s the final meta-analysis conclusions have been cautiously interp[reted] [A] s a US Food and Drug Administration–approved modality; how[ever] [r]emains strictly off-label.

Dev[ices]

[Tr]anspyloric shuttle

[Tr]anspyloric shuttle (TPS; Baronova, Goleta, CA) is a non-su[rgical] [u]ses a large spherical proximal silicone bulb attached with a [cyli]ndrical bulb. The device is deployed into the stomach vi[a] [syst]em that incorporates a flexible introducer sheath throug[h] [pa]ssed in elongated form. The TPS device assembles a[t] [whic]h, consisting of a smooth outer skin into which the inte[rnal] [a]nd is locked. The device is delivered to the stomach, [With] [p]eristalsis, the distal cylindrical bulb (about the size o[f] such as sodium morrhuate into the GJ aperture, thereby creating submucosal blebs, which reduce stomal diameter, initially through edema and later by fibrosis following inflammation. In 2003, 20 patients with a dilated GJ stoma underwent sclerotherapy with sodium morrhuate.[16] The study demonstrated a good safety profile, technical feasibility, and results, noting GJ stomal reduction to 9 to 10 mm after an average of 1.3 sessions. Twelve-month follow-up data revealed that 91.6% of patients achieved persistent weight loss or weight stabilization after sclerotherapy. Subsequent observational studies have reiterated persistent weight loss or weight regain stabilization after endoscopic sclerotherapy.[17–19] A 2012 large retrospective study, summarizing 231 patients, revealed that 78% of study patients experienced weight-regain stabilization at 12 months after the procedure.[20]

Although there may be more effective methods of managing after-RYGB weight gain, endoscopic sclerotherapy is a straightforward, cost-effective, minimally invasive, technically facile procedure that can be used by the general gastroenterologist or surgeon. Given the positive outcomes in the literature related to after-RYGB stomal sclerotherapy, this would seem a legitimate therapeutic option to ameliorate after-RYGB weight regain.

Endoscopic radiofrequency ablation

Radiofrequency ablation (RFA) therapy represents direct thermal energy administration to gastrointestinal mucosal tissue. Serial RFA ablation of the after-RYGB gastric pouch and GJ aperture may alter pouch compliance, aperture diameter, and gastric wall compliance, which could produce early satiety and subsequent weight loss. A 2016 prospective multicentered pilot study was performed to further qualify the weight loss potential of the RFA device.[21] Twenty-five subjects with documented weight regain after RYGB were enrolled in the trial. These subjects had to have lost 40% of their excess weight postoperatively and then regained 25% back. At 12-month follow-up, and after up to 3 treatment sessions done at 4-month intervals, the mean post-RFA excess body weight loss was reported at 30.4%. Adverse events were reported in 40% of patients, with complaints often related to abdominal pain and vomiting. The initial results are encouraging, albeit with significant transient postprocedural discomfort. Larger studies, including sham-controlled ones, will be required to fully characterize the benefits of the RFA device for post–gastric bypass weight regain and to define the mechanism of effect, such as altered gastric wall compliance, signaling, stomal emptying, or other treatment result.

Gastric Volume Restriction Devices

Transoral endoscopic restrictive implant system device

The transoral endoscopic restrictive implant system (TERIS) device (BaroSense, Redwood, CA) consisted of an endoscopically placed restrictive silicone diaphragm with a 10-mm orifice that was anchored in the gastric cardia with transmural plications. The gastric plications were performed by a novel independently functional endoscopic stapling device. The TERIS system created a luminal stenosis just distal to the gastroesophageal (GE) junction in the gastric cardia. The acquired anatomy after the procedure essentially mimics the laparoscopic-assisted gastric banding (LAGB) surgery.

The device was developed and refined with the use of the canine animal model. Canine gastric tissue was thought to best approximate human gastric tissue and aided in the device-testing process of the tissue plication technology. More than 200 canines were used for device development, with no reported severe adverse events.

The TERIS procedure was initiated with a 5-mm gastroscope and stapling device, both of which were advanced simultaneously via an overtube. The stapler is directed to the gastric cardia mucosa roughly 3 cm distal to the GE junction. The stapler has a suction port that helps to acquire, compress, and facilitate full-thickness transmural plication. Five total transmural plications are performed. Through a series of complex maneuvers, respective silicone membranes were deployed at the plication sites with corresponding anchors. The silicone diaphragm implant was then fastened to the gastric cardia anchors to complete device placement. Follow-up diaphragm removal was performed with the assistance of a gastroscope. The anchor heads were endoscopically visualized, and an internal cutting snare was used to cut each anchor. The diaphragm was subsequently removed via the overtube.

A large phase I observational human clinical trial was performed to further investigate the device.[22] During enrollment, there were 3 complications within the first 7 patients, including 2 cases of pneumoperitoneum and one case of gastric perforation. Procedural adjustments were made including switching from air insufflation to carbon dioxide and performing staple plications 1 cm distal to the original plication sites. Thirteen patients ultimately enrolled, and following procedural adjustments, major adverse events were eliminated. Three-month follow-up revealed a mean EWL of 28%. The observed weight loss response is similar to the cited 3-month after-LAGB follow-up outcome data.[23]

A 2016 follow-up study of the aforementioned patient cohort was performed. The study population consisted of 18 patients, and the mean EWL was 30.1% at 6 months.[24] The results demonstrate that the TERIS system had significant weight loss potential. However, at 6-month follow-up endoscopy, the anchors remained intact in only 62.5% of patients, which raised concerns regarding device durability. Ultimately, the initial complications, procedural complexity, and the lack of device durability led to cessation of the clinical trial and abandonment of further TERIS device development.

Articulating circular endoscopic stapler

The articulating circular endoscopic (ACE) stapler (Boston Scientific Corporation, Natick, MA) is a full-thickness stapling device system with the flexibility of 360° stapling. This stapler device was originally used in the now defunct TERIS system and now acquired by Boston Scientific.

From a procedural standpoint, the ACE stapler has the ability to retroflex, to use a suctioning port to acquire tissue, and to deploy full-thickness tissue staples to plicate redundant gastric tissue. Serial plications throughout the stomach lead to restricted gastric volume, which in theory should promote weight loss. Preclinical animal model data demonstrated a good safety profile without adverse events.

A phase I observational human pilot study was performed in the Netherlands. The 17-patient study revealed a mean 34.9% EWL at 12-month follow-up.[25] On average, 8 staples were placed in the fundus, and 2 staples in the antrum. Upper endoscopy at the end of the study revealed 6 to 9 plications in place with preserved reduced gastric volume in all 17 patients. Transient self-resolving abdominal pain, nausea, and vomiting were reported after the procedure. This pilot study demonstrates procedural feasibility with a good safety profile in both the short and the long term. A 24-month follow-up study is currently underway.

A 2013 DDW (Digestive Disease Week) abstract evaluated gastric physiology after ACE stapling.[26] Results noted that at 1-month follow-up, there was evidence of significant weight loss, reduced caloric intake, and increased patient reported satiety. There were no significant changes in gastric emptying as evidenced by follow-up emptying scans.

FullSense device

The FullSense device (Sentinel Group, Grand Rapids, MI) is a stent-type device consisting of a proximal esophageal component linked to a distal gastric one, which puts

Selected Endoscopic Gastric Devices for Obesity

 CrossMark

Kartik Sampath, MD*, Richard I. Rothstein, MD

KEYWORDS

- Obesity • Stomach • Bariatric endoscopy • Therapeutic endoscopy • Devices

KEY POINTS

- Endoscopic devices can treat obesity and its related metabolic conditions by targeting key gastric anatomic and physiologic mechanisms.
- Recognizing the effect of the bariatric surgical interventions on gastric anatomy and physiology will contribute to the development of minimally invasive devices that can mimic these effects.
- There are many bariatric endoscopic devices, in various stages of development, targeting the stomach to promote caloric restriction and early satiety through anatomic and physiologic effects.
- The Transpyloric Shuttle involves several mechanisms of action, including occupying space, blocking the gastric exit, delaying gastric emptying, and potentially altering hormonal signaling.
- Gastric sclerotherapy, Botulinum toxin A injection, and radiofrequency ablation likely change gastric or postoperative stomal compliance or motility and emptying physiology and have been shown to produce weight loss. The ACE stapler represents a novel gastric volume-reducing device; further clinical study is needed.
- The Gelesis100 device and the Magnetic Weight Loss Capsule represent applications of material science and mechanical engineering, and with further study, can open avenues of clinical application.
- Randomized, blinded controlled trials are needed to determine the true effect of these unique devices beyond sham.

Financial Disclosures: Dr R.I. Rothstein has received research grant support from BaroNova (NCT02518685) and Barrx/Medtronic (NCT01910688) as well as consulting fees from Boston Scientific. He is on the scientific advisory board of Allurion.
Section of Gastroenterology and Hepatology, Department of Medicine, Dartmouth-Hitchcock Medical Center, Geisel School of Medicine at Dartmouth, One Medical Center Drive, Lebanon, NH 03756, USA
* Corresponding author.
E-mail address: kartik.sampath@hitchcock.org

SELECTED STOMACH TARGET DEVICES
Introduction

The obesity epidemic refers to the rising incidence of obesity worldwide and its impact on global health.[1] Bariatric surgery remains the most effective therapeutic option for obesity. At present, the overwhelming demand far exceeds the health care infrastructure capable of providing bariatric surgical services. Endoscopic therapy for obesity represents a potentially cost-effective, accessible, minimally invasive alternative that can function as both a primary therapeutic intervention and a bridge to bariatric surgery.

Endoscopic devices that target the stomach directly alter gastric physiology and promote weight loss by altering functional gastric volume, gastric emptying, gastric wall compliance, neurohormonal signaling, and satiety. Intragastric balloons (IGBs) and the endoscopic sleeve gastroplasty (ESG) procedure restrict functional gastric volume, which causes decreased caloric intake, increased satiety, and eventual weight loss. Aspiration therapy (AT) removes excess caloric ingestion directly from the stomach via an aspiration tube upon initial food bolus ingestion. These devices, in particular, are discussed extensively in separate respective articles. This article focuses on the non-IGB, non-ESG, non-AT stomach target devices that are currently in various stages of development and offer promise for future weight loss therapies.

It is important to understand the basic gastric physiology and motility, and the physiologic alterations of the bariatric surgical procedures, when evaluating the role and utility of current and future bariatric devices that target the stomach. With food ingestion, gastric accommodation initially produces fundic and corpus relaxation, with concurrent pyloric contraction and closure. The result is food bolus accumulation in the stomach. The mixing stage represents vagal nerve–mediated gastric antral contractions, which churn the food bolus against a contracted pylorus, with trituration of the ingesta. The emptying phase refers to pyloric relaxation with continued antral pump contraction. The food bolus then passes into the duodenum for further digestion and absorption. Neurohormonal signaling plays an instrumental role during the entire gastric digestive process. The integrated signaling that occurs with the act of eating, and through the process of gastric accommodation and emptying, has a complex interplay for the sensation of satiety and hunger and regulates processes that relate to energy balance, obesity, and related metabolic disorders. Understanding how medical and surgical bariatric interventions affect these mechanisms can direct the development of effective endoscopic devices. These devices may target anatomic processes and result in restriction of caloric intake or produce mal-digestion. It is likely that devices that will be most effective and durable will be ones that alter physiologic mechanisms, and much study is still needed to identify the changes that these devices may produce and which ones will be efficacious and safe. With other contributions detailing what is known about the currently approved gastric devices and techniques, and additional ones highlighting emerging new therapies, the authors focus on the remaining devices or techniques not covered elsewhere in this issue.

Devices/Techniques Affecting Gastric Emptying

Gastric botulinum toxin A injection

Botulinum toxin A (BTA) is an acetylcholinesterase inhibitor that functions as a long-acting inhibitor of both voluntary and smooth muscle contraction leading to a reversible paralytic-type effect. Direct injection into the gastric antral smooth muscle offers the potential to delay gastric emptying by moderating the propulsive contraction effect of the antral pump. In theory, pump inhibition leads to impaired gastric emptying, increased satiety, inhibition of ghrelin release, decreased oral intake, and eventual weight loss.

Preclinical animal studies were initially performed in rats. In 2000, a prospective, 3-way parallel, randomized controlled study was performed whereby rats were subjected to laparotomy with gastric BTA injection, sham laparotomy, or control group without laparotomy.[2] At 10-week follow-up, there was significant weight loss in the BTA group versus the sham group (14.0% vs 4.4% [maximum weight loss as a percentage], $P<.001$). In 2005, a follow-up randomized, sham-controlled study in a specific obese rat population, reiterated findings of significant weight loss in the BTA injection group.[3]

Numerous human pilot studies were subsequently performed. In 2005, an 8-patient observational study demonstrated feasibility and safety of the gastric BTA injection method.[4] During a standard upper endoscopy, BTA was directly injected into the antral mucosa. Compared with baseline patient weights, there was a significant mean weight reduction at 1 month after BTA (121.8 kg vs 124.6 kg, $P<.05$). Further pilot studies investigated optimal BTA dosing administrations, and BTA effects on gastric emptying; however, the results were generally equivocal.[5,6]

In 2007, a randomized, sham-controlled study with 6-month follow-up revealed weight reduction that was not statistically significant in the BTA group.[7] Conversely, a randomized controlled trial, performed in 2012, administered BTA injections throughout the stomach including the fundus.[8] The results noted statistically significant weight loss at the interval 12-week follow-up.

In 2007, a randomized, sham-controlled trial revealed significant weight loss (11.0 vs 5.7 kg, $P<.001$) and body mass index (BMI) reduction (4.00 vs 2.00 kg/m^2, $P<.001$) in the BTA group during 12-week follow-up.[9] This study was noteworthy for also demonstrating significantly decreased gastric-emptying time in the BTA group ($+18.9$ vs -2.2, $P<.05$).

Given the equivocal data regarding mucosal-based gastric BTA injection therapy, studies investigated submucosal BTA injection into the muscularis propria. In 2008, a pilot study was performed via endoscopic ultrasound–guided BTA injections into the antral submucosa. At 16-week follow-up, the average body weight loss was 4.9 (±6.3) kg.[10] A follow-up double-blinded, randomized, sham-controlled trial was conducted in 2013.[11] At 24-week follow-up, there was no significant weight loss; however, significantly delayed gastric emptying was observed in the 300-unit BTA injection cohort.

A 2015 meta-analysis was performed summarizing the 8 gastric BTA studies to date, 5 of which were randomized controlled trials. The results did reveal statistically significant weight loss effects with gastric BTA treatment.[12] A follow-up editorial reviewing the study raised concerns regarding the study methodology, particularly the inclusion of non-randomized controlled trials in statistical subanalysis. As a result, the final meta-analysis conclusions have been cautiously interpreted.[13] Currently, BTA is a US Food and Drug Administration–approved modality; however, its use for obesity remains strictly off-label.

Transpyloric shuttle

Transpyloric shuttle (TPS; Baronova, Goleta, CA) is a non-surgical device that comprises a large spherical proximal silicone bulb attached with a tether to a smaller distal cylindrical bulb. The device is deployed into the stomach via an integrated delivery system that incorporates a flexible introducer sheath through which the TPS device is passed in elongated form. The TPS device assembles at the end of the delivery sheath, consisting of a smooth outer skin into which the internal silicone component coils and is locked. The device is delivered to the stomach, and with normal physiologic peristalsis, the distal cylindrical bulb (about the size of a large olive) advances to the proximal duodenum. The tether traverses the pylorus, and the larger spherical bulb remains positioned in the antrum. The larger bulb intermittently engages the pylorus during peristalsis, leading to transient gastric outlet obstruction, but then falls back into the stomach, allowing for gastric content to pass through the pylorus intermittently, hence the "shuttle" effect. In the clinical trials to date, the device placement is for 6 to 12 months, followed by mandatory removal. Retrieval of the device requires the use of a modified standard esophageal overtube using rat-tooth graspers and a snare to unlock and uncoil the components of the proximal bulb, removing them through the overtube and then grasping the outer skin and removing it from the stomach.

The TPS has several key mechanisms of action that promote weight loss. The large bulb, although not sized as much as the water- or gas-filled balloons, represents a space-occupying device, similar to IGBs, which partially reduces functional gastric volume. During antral contractions, the large bulb repeatedly engages the pylorus, causing intermittent obstruction. This action delays gastric emptying, prolongs gastric accommodation, and increases satiety. It is possible that the distal bulb is interacting with duodenal mucosa and incretin signaling, although this remains to be elucidated.

In 2014, a prospective, nonrandomized single-center clinical trial reported the feasibility, safety, and efficacy of the TPS device.[14] A total of 20 patients were enrolled, all of which had a BMI between 30 and 50 kg/m^2. Proton pump inhibitors were administered for all patients during the length of the study. The device was safely deployed and removed in all 20 patients. At 3- and 6-month follow-up, 25.1% and 44.0% excess weight loss (EWL) were observed, respectively. Ninety percent of study patients revealed maximum weight loss at the time of device removal, which suggested the possibility of longer-term weight loss potential. Two patients required early device removal due to gastric ulceration.

Following strong pilot data, the pivotal ENDObesity II study was initiated in the United States, which represents a multicenter, randomized, sham-controlled clinical trial. The target study population (n = 270, 2:1 randomization for the device) includes patients who have failed lifestyle changes or medical therapy, with a BMI of 30.0 to 40.0. The study has completed subject enrollment, with early observation being highly encouraging for safely producing weight loss.

The TPS device is designed for temporary placement and does not fundamentally alter the gastrointestinal anatomy. Similar to IGBs, the indications for TPS placement may be both for primary obesity management and as a bridge to bariatric surgery. This device may also prove to be useful for the pediatric population. In addition to defining the weight loss potential, translational research studies investigating the corresponding neurohormonal signaling are warranted to better characterize the antiobesity effects of the TPS device.

Devices/Techniques Affecting Gastric Wall or Postbypass Stomal Compliance

Endoscopic sclerotherapy

As prefaced in the article dedicated to endoscopic revision of Roux-en-Y gastric bypass (RYGB), weight regain after bariatric surgery is a common complication. Acquired anatomic defects can contribute to weight regain, including gastric-gastric fistula and dilated gastrojejunal (GJ) anastomosis. GJ aperture reduction has been shown to curb weight regain and promote weight loss by potentially delaying gastric emptying and increasing satiety.[15]

An option to alter compliance of the postbypass stoma and thereby effect weight loss by altering the kinetics of emptying may be accomplished with the use of endoscopic sclerotherapy. Endoscopic sclerotherapy involves the injection of a sclerosant pressure on these areas. There was resultant production of satiety and weight loss in a pilot trial conducted in Mexico with implant duration of 6 weeks.[27] Subjects safely lost weight until the devices were removed, with resultant weight regain with devices removed. No publications are available for review of clinical experience.

Gelesis100 hydrogel capsule

Gelesis100 (Gelesis, Boston, MA) is a swallowable capsule that contains thousands of tiny hydrogel particles and is designed to follow the natural food cycle. The particles consist of modified cellulose strands crosslinked to one another by citric acid. The resultant composition is a hydrophilic lattice network that absorbs water and rapidly expands. Water absorption increases each particle size by 100-fold, and the external particle layer continues to maintain inherent structural integrity and elasticity, which precludes coalescence with extraneous food particles.

Capsule ingestion occurs prior to a meal and is accompanied by water. Upon entering the stomach, the capsule dissolves, allowing hydrogel particles to interact with water and expand. The expanded particles essentially create a temporary space occupying "device", thereby reducing gastric volume for caloric intake. As the Gelesis100 particles advance into the duodenum, the luminal contents are more viscous. The particles provide a pseudo-barrier that impairs total glucose absorption and may in theory improve glycemic control. Gelesis100 particles eventually breaks down in the large intestine with colonic water resorption leading to hydrogel excretion.

A 2014 study investigated the therapeutic utility of the Gelesis100 device in a double-blinded randomized placebo controlled study in human subjects. One hundred twenty-eight nondiabetic overweight patients were randomized to a 3-arm study, including Gelesis 2.25 g twice daily versus Gelesis 3.75 g twice daily versus placebo over a 12-week period.[28] The intention-to-treat analysis revealed statistically significant weight loss in the 2.25-g treatment arm compared with placebo (6.1 vs 4.1% weight reduction, $P = .026$). The investigators suggest that tolerability and compliance issues with the 3.75-g treatment arm may have led to the surprisingly lower observed weight loss. The device demonstrated a good safety profile with no major adverse events. Given the strong study design, the results are encouraging. However, longer-term data are needed to further validate this technology.

Magnetically weight loss capsule

IGBs, depending on the type, are often placed and removed endoscopically. These requirements increase general health costs as well as patient morbidity related to sedation and endoscopy. A novel IGB known as the magnetically weight loss capsule (MWLC) is delivered as a swallowable capsule and uses magnet technology to activate balloon inflation and deflation.[29] The device currently is in the developmental stage and has been trialed ex vivo in the porcine stomach. The magnetic capsule balloon is ingested with a glass of water. Once the capsule reaches the stomach, a properly oriented magnet is externally placed on the subject's stomach, which activates balloon inflation. Reversing the external magnet orientation causes balloon deflation. Once deflated, the balloon can safely pass, in theory, per rectum. The major potential benefits relate to the elimination of endoscopy for capsule placement and removal.

The capsule consists of 2 chambers containing citric acid and potassium bicarbonate, respectively, separated by an inflation valve and 2 internal magnets. The extracorporeal magnet can orient the capsule to open the inflation valve and promote acid-base mixture, resulting in carbon dioxide gas production and balloon inflation. Conversely, reversing external magnet polarity will preclude mixing and allow balloon gas extrusion. At this time, the designed prototype capsule is a latex balloon, which is a material prone to rupture. The balloon size is 170 mL, which is considerably smaller than current commercial balloons. Revised magnet actuated capsule development will undoubtedly be necessary. However, as a proof of concept study, the MWLC represents an exciting first step, and a potentially promising future antiobesity device.

SUMMARY

This brief review addressed the endoscopic devices that target the stomach and for the most part were not covered in other contributions in this issue. There is a spectrum of device development, from promising start-up ideas, to strong preliminary preclinical experience, to variable but often positive initial clinical trial outcomes, as well as some admirably failed ventures. Gastric function continues to remain an exceedingly interesting and complex mechanical and physiologic process. Targeting devices that affect and alter foregut anatomic and physiologic functions, with mimicry of the current effective bariatric surgical procedures, will produce techniques and treatments with safe and effective antiobesity profiles. With continued preclinical device development and well-designed clinical trials with standardized outcome metrics, there is the potential to identify the key devices that best modulate these processes and achieve the optimal weight loss outcomes.

REFERENCES

1. James WP. WHO recognition of the global obesity epidemic. Int J Obes (Lond) 2008;32(Suppl 7):S120–6. Review.
2. Gui D, de Gaetano A, Spada PL, et al. Botulinum toxin injected in the gastric wall reduces body weight and food intake in rats. Aliment Pharmacol Ther 2000;14(6): 829–34.
3. Coskun H, Duran Y, Dilege E, et al. Effect on gastric emptying and weight reduction of botulinum toxin-A injection into the gastric antral layer: an experimental study in the obese rat model. Obes Surg 2005;15:1137–43.
4. Albani G, Petroni ML, Mauro A, et al. Safety and efficacy of therapy with botulinum toxin in obesity: a pilot study. J Gastroenterol 2005;40(8):833–5.
5. Júnior AC, Savassi-Rocha PR, Coelho LG, et al. Botulinum A toxin injected into the gastric wall for the treatment of class III obesity: a pilot study. Obes Surg 2006;16(3):335–43.
6. Gui D, Mingrone G, Valenza V, et al. Effect of botulinum toxin antral injection on gastric emptying and weight reduction in obese patients: a pilot study. Aliment Pharmacol Ther 2006;23:675–80.
7. Mittermair R, Keller C, Geibel J. Intragastric injection of botulinum toxin A for the treatment of obesity. Obes Surg 2007;17:732–6.
8. Li L, Liu Q-S, Liu W-H, et al. Treatment of obesity by endoscopic gastric intramural injection of botulinum toxin A: a randomized clinical trial. Hepatogastroenterology 2012;59(118):2003–7.
9. Foschi D, Corsi F, Lazzaroni M, et al. Treatment of morbid obesity by intraparietogastric administration of botulinum toxin: a randomized, double-blind, controlled study. Int J Obes 2007;31:707–12.
10. Topazian M, Camilleri M, De La Mora-Levy J, et al. Endoscopic ultrasound-guided gastric botulinum toxin injections in obese subjects: a pilot study. Obes Surg 2008;18(4):401–7.
11. Topazian M, Camilleri M, Enders FT, et al. Gastric antral injections of botulinum toxin delay gastric emptying but do not reduce body weight. Clin Gastroenterol Hepatol 2013;11(2):145–50.

12. Bang CS, Baik GH, Shin IS, et al. Effect of intragastric injection of botulinum toxin A for the treatment of obesity: a meta-analysis and meta-regression. Gastrointest Endosc 2015;81(5):1141–9.

13. de Moura EG, Bustamante FA, Bernardo WM. Reviewing the reviewers: critical appraisal of "Effect of intragastric injection of botulinum toxin A for the treatment of obesity: a meta-analysis and meta-regression". Gastrointest Endosc 2016;83(2):478.

14. Marinos G, Eliades C, Raman Muthusamy V, et al. Weight loss and improved quality of life with a nonsurgical endoscopic treatment for obesity: clinical results from a 3- and 6-month study. Surg Obes Relat Dis 2014;10(5):929–34.

15. Jirapinyo P, Slattery J, Ryan MB, et al. Evaluation of an endoscopic suturing device for transoral outlet reduction in patients with weight regain following Roux-en-Y gastric bypass. Endoscopy 2013;45(7):532–6.

16. Spaulding L. Treatment of dilated gastrojejunostomy with sclerotherapy. Obes Surg 2003;13:254–7.

17. Spaulding L, Osler T, Patlak J. Long-term results of sclerotherapy for dilated gastrojejunostomy after gastric bypass. Surg Obes Relat Dis 2007;3(6):623–6.

18. Loewen M, Barba C. Endoscopic sclerotherapy for dilated gastrojejunostomy of failed gastric bypass. Surg Obes Relat Dis 2008;4(4):539–42.

19. Giurgius M, Fearing N, Weir A, et al. Long-term follow-up evaluation of endoscopic sclerotherapy for dilated gastrojejunostomy after gastric bypass. Surg Endosc 2014;28(5):1454–9.

20. Abu Dayyeh BK, Jirapinyo P, Weitzner Z, et al. Endoscopic sclerotherapy for the treatment of weight regain after Roux-en-Y gastric bypass: outcomes, complications, and predictors of response in 575 procedures. Gastrointest Endosc 2012;76(2):275–82.

21. Abrams JA, Komanduri S, Shaheen N, et al. Radiofrequency ablation for the treatment of weight regain after roux-en-y gastric bypass. Gastroenterology 2016;150(4):S824.

22. de Jong K, Mathus-Vliegen EM, Veldhuyzen EA, et al. Short-term safety and efficacy of the Trans-oral Endoscopic Restrictive Implant System for the treatment of obesity. Gastrointest Endosc 2010;72(3):497–504.

23. Jan JC, Hong D, Pereira N, et al. Laparoscopic adjustable gastric banding versus laparoscopic gastric bypass for morbid obesity: a single-institution comparison study of early results. J Gastrointest Surg 2005;9(1):30–9 [discussion: 40–1].

24. Verlaan T, de Jong K, de la Mar-Ploem ED, et al. Trans-oral Endoscopic Restrictive Implant System: endoscopic treatment of obesity? Surg Obes Relat Dis 2016;12(9):1711–8.

25. Verlaan T, Paulus GF, Mathus-Vliegen EM. Endoscopic gastric volume reduction with a novel articulating plication device is safe and effective in the treatment of obesity (with video). Gastrointest Endosc 2015;81(2):312–20.

26. Avesaat MV, Paulus GF, Conchillo JM, et al. First Results of the Barosense ACE Stapler Procedure for the treatment of morbid obesity: effect on food intake and satiety. Gastroenterology 2013;144(5):S320.

27. Available at: http://www.biomedicine.org/medicine-news-1/weight-loss-without-hunger-21-36609-1/.Accessed November 30, 2016.

28. Arne A, Mette K, Lucio G. Oral Administration of Gelesis100, a novel hydrogel, significantly decreases body weight in overweight and obese subjects. Available at: http://www.gelesis.com/pdf/Handout_EndocrineSociety2014.pdf. Accessed November 28, 2016.

29. Do TN, Seah TE, Ho KY, et al. Development and testing of a magnetically actuated capsule endoscopy for obesity treatment. PLoS One 2016;11(1):e0148035.

Aspiration Therapy for Obesity

Shelby Sullivan, MD

KEYWORDS

- Aspiration therapy • Endoscopic bariatric therapy • AspireAssist

KEY POINTS

- The AspireAssist System was recently approved by the Food and Drug Administration (FDA) to perform aspiration therapy.
- Aspiration therapy removes up to 30% of calories consumed at a meal but also induces a decrease in food intake and improved eating behaviors.
- Percent total body weight loss (%TBWL) across trials in patients completing 52 weeks of therapy is 14.2% to 21.4%.
- Serious adverse event (SAE) rates are low, no deaths have occurred, and no patients have developed binge eating disorder or bulimia as a result of aspiration therapy.

INTRODUCTION

One of the key components in the pathophysiology of obesity is the intake of calories in excess of energy expenditure resulting in storage of energy, mainly in the form of triglycerides. The physiologic control of eating by the adipose tissue–gut–brain axis has been extensively studied.[1] Humans eat for a variety of reasons, however, including hedonic likability of food, social influences, emotional stress, and environmental cues that are less well understood and may over-ride physiologic mechanisms for appetite regulation.[2] Moreover, lifestyle interventions aimed at modifying behaviors related to these psychosocial factors yield only modest weight loss.[3] Aspiration therapy, an endoscopic bariatric therapy (EBT) that removes up to 30% of calories in a meal, may overcome the limitations of lifestyle intervention alone in reducing food intake to level required for greater weight loss. This review details aspiration therapy with the recently FDA-approved AspireAssist System (Aspire Bariatrics, King of Prussia, Pennsylvania).

Contracted Research for ReShape Medical, GI Dynamics, Aspire Bariatrics, USGI Medical, Obalon Therapeutics, BARonova, Paion; consultant for USGI Medical, Obalon, SynerZ, and Elira Therapeutics.
Department of Internal Medicine, University of Colorado School of Medicine, Mail Stop B158 Academic Office 1, 12631 East 17th Avenue, Aurora, CO 80045, USA
E-mail address: shelby.sullivan@ucdenver.edu

Gastrointest Endoscopy Clin N Am 27 (2017) 277–288
http://dx.doi.org/10.1016/j.giec.2016.12.001
giendo.theclinics.com

ASPIRATION AND THE COMPONENTS OF THE AspireAssist SYSTEM

Aspiration therapy involves the aspiration of gastric contents after a meal to reduce total calorie absorption for weight loss. The therapy requires the use of the AspireAssist System, which is seen in **Fig. 1** and described.

Permanent Components

- A-Tube: a 42-cm silicone tube attached to a dilator and metal cable loop used to attach the A-Tube to a flexible guide wire for placement through the abdominal wall with the standard pull percutaneous endoscopic gastrostomy (PEG) tube technique (see **Fig. 1**A).[4] After implantation, the delivery tube portion of the A-Tube with the dilator and metal loop are cut and discarded. The remaining A-Tube has an intragastric bumper that prevents migration through the gastrocutaneous tract. Unlike a standard PEG tube, the A-Tube also contains a 15-cm intragastric portion lined with fenestrations to facilitate the flow of gastric contents into the A-tube.
- Skin-Port: a 3.5-cm disk with a height of less than 1 cm, which is connected to the external portion of the A-Tube. The Skin-Port contains a valve that can be opened to allow gastric contents to flow out when opened with the Connector (discussed later)

Components Only Attached During Aspiration

- Connector: a disk that attaches to the Skin-Port and opens the valve in the Skin-Port (see **Fig. 1**B). The Connector also contains a counter that tracks the number of times the Skin-Port is opened. After 115 uses, or the equivalent of 5 weeks to 6 weeks of therapy, the Connector locks and can no longer be used to open the Skin-Port.
- Patient Line: a flexible silicone tube that connects the Connector to the Companion (discussed later)
- Companion: a passive siphon with that allows for flow of water into the Patient Line through the Connector into the A-Tube to facilitate aspiration of gastric contents and flow of gastric contents out of the stomach into the Patient Line and out of the Companion
- Reservoir: a 600-mL soft water bottle that can be filled with tap water and attaches to the Companion to infuse into the stomach to facilitate aspiration of gastric contents
- Drain Tube: silicone tube that attaches to the bottom of the Companion and provides a clean exit of gastric contents into the toilet

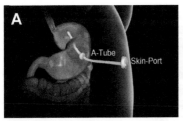
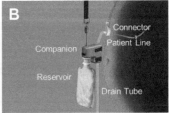

Fig. 1. Components of the AspireAssist System: (*A*) permanent components and (*B*) components only used during aspiration.

PATIENT EVALUATION OVERVIEW

The indications for use of the AspireAssist System as listed in the FDA Summary of Safety and Effectiveness Data document,[5] include patients age 22 and older with a body mass index (BMI) of 35.0 kg/m^2 to 55.0 kg/m^2 who have not been able to lose or maintain a weight loss with nonsurgical weight loss therapy. The FDA summary specifically includes lifestyle therapy and continuous medical monitoring as components of the AspireAssist System. These are consistent with medical society position statements, which confirm that EBTs are intended to be used in conjunction with a lifestyle therapy program and medical monitoring.[6]

Contraindications for use are listed in **Box 1**. Most contraindications can be determined by standard medical history and physical examination, laboratory evaluation, or endoscopy. Diagnosing bulimia, binge eating disorder, or night eating syndrome using *Diagnostic and Statistical Manual of Mental Disorders* (Fifth Edition) (*DSM-5*) criteria[7] may pose more of a challenge to endoscopists who likely have not been trained in making these diagnoses. The FDA does not require patients to be seen by a psychologist for evaluation; however, the author suggests that if patients exhibit signs of an eating disorder on history or on eating disorder questionnaires, referral should be made to a psychologist or psychiatrist with expertise in eating disorders. The most common questionnaire assessments of eating behaviors used in the preoperative

---

Box 1
Contraindications for use of the AspireAssist System

Previous abdominal surgery that increases the risk of gastrostomy tube placement

Esophageal stricture, pseudo-obstruction, severe gastroparesis, gastric outlet obstruction

Inflammatory bowel disease

History of refractory gastric ulcers

Ulcers, bleeding lesions, or tumors discovered during endoscopic examination

Uncontrolled hypertension (blood pressure >160/100 mm Hg)

History or evidence of serious pulmonary or cardiovascular disease (acute coronary syndrome, New York Heart Association class III or IV heart failure

Coagulation disorder (platelets <50,000, prothrombin time >2 seconds above control or international normalized ratio >1.5)

Anemia (hemoglobin <8.0 g/dL in women and <10.0 g/dL in men)

Pregnancy or lactation

Diagnosed bulimia or diagnosed binge eating disorder using *DSM-5* criteria

Night eating syndrome

Chronic abdominal pain that potentially complicates the management of the device

Physical or mental disability or psychologic illness that could interfere with the compliance of therapy

At high risk for having a medical complication from the endoscopic procedure or the AspireAssist weight loss program for any reason, including general poor health or severe organ dysfunction, such as cirrhosis or renal dysfunction

From FDA. Summary of safety and effectiveness data (SSED) AspireAssist. In: FDA, editor. 2016. p. 1–36.

bariatric surgical patient,[8] which are also appropriate for preprocedural aspiration therapy patients, include

- Questionnaire on Eating and Weight Patterns-5[9]
- Three-Factor Eating Questionnaire[10]
- Eating Disorder Examination Questionnaire[11]
- Binge Eating Scale[12]

In addition to the FDA-labeled contraindications, treating physicians should review the requirements for successful aspiration therapy prior to device placement. Patients need the flexibility to be able to go to a restroom or other facility where they are able to perform aspiration 20 minutes after a meal. Total time for aspiration, including set-up and clean-up, takes 10 minutes to 15 minutes on average. Patients who are unable to reliably perform aspiration are not likely to achieve significant weight loss.

OUTCOMES
Weight Loss

Four studies have investigated the effects of aspiration therapy one weight loss in subjects with a BMI between 35 kg/m^2 and 55 kg/m^2:

- Mexico pilot study: 26-week pilot study in Mexico[13]
- US pilot study: 52-week randomized controlled pilot trial in the United States[14]
- Swedish pilot study: 26-week pilot trial in Sweden[15]
- Pivotal Aspiration Therapy with Adjusted Lifestyle Therapy Study (PATHWAY): 52-week multicenter randomized controlled trial in the United States[16]

Additionally, 1 multicenter European trial evaluated the effects of aspiration therapy on subjects with a BMI greater than 55 kg/m^2 (European superobesity pilot study).[17] Details of subject characteristics are in **Table 1**. The Mexico pilot study and part of the US pilot study were performed with the first generation of the AspireAssist System. The major difference between the first-generation and second-generation devices is the A-Tube. The extragastric portion of the original A-Tube was made of an expanded polytetrafluoroethylene (ePTFE) tube and was reinforced with a helical ePTFE wire with the intragastric portion made of silicone. The redesign to the all-silicone tube occurred during the US pilot trial in response to patient discomfort with the ePTFE portion of the A-Tube.

Weight loss details of these trials are in **Table 2**. Each of the studies allowed subjects to continue therapy after the prespecified protocol was complete. Available data on weight loss in subjects who continued beyond the prespecified study duration are listed where available. The BMI 35 kg/m^2 to 55 kg/m^2 studies were consistent in ratio of men to women, average age, average weight, and average BMI. More men than women enrolled in the BMI greater than 55 kg/m^2 trial, and, as expected, both weight and BMI were significantly higher than in the BMI 35 kg/m^2 to 55 kg/m^2 trials. Weight loss in both the US pilot study and PATHWAY was higher in the aspiration therapy groups compared with the control groups receiving lifestyle therapy only ($P = .021$ and $P<.01$, respectively). Additionally, weight loss in subjects who completed 52 weeks of therapy in the PATHWAY was closer to the previously published pilot trials in the United States and Sweden, with %TBWL of 4.9% $\pm$ 7.0% in the control group (n = 31) and 14.2% $\pm$ 9.8% in the aspiration therapy group (n = 82; $P<.01$). These data suggest that %TBWL with aspiration therapy in conjunction with lifestyle therapy is 2.9 to 3.2 times more effective than lifestyle therapy alone. In addition, weight loss is consistent across different cultures and a wide range of BMI.

Table 1
Characteristics of subjects in studies evaluating aspiration therapy

Study Group	Number (Male/Female)	Age (y)	Weight (kg)	Body Mass Index (kg/m^2)
Mexico pilot study[13],[a]	9 (0/9)	41.6 ± 0.1	110.1 ± 14.9	40.0 ± 3.1
US pilot study control group[a]	4 (1/3)	45.3 ± 2.8	105.3 ± 2.5	39.3 ± 1.1
US pilot study aspiration therapy group[a]	10 (0/10)	38.7 ± 2.3	112.2 ± 4.6	42.0 ± 1.4
Sweden pilot study[a]	22 (2/20)	49.8 ± 7.7	109.8 ± 18.6	40.3 ± 4.3
PATHWAY control group	60 (7/53)	46.8 ± 11.6	112.8 ± 16.1	40.9 ± 3.9
PATHWAY aspiration therapy group	111 (15/96)	42.4 ± 10.0	116.9 ± 21.2	42.0 ± 5.1
European superobesity pilot study	11 (8/3)	44.9 (32–63)	196.1 (143.0–290.0)	66.5 (55.0–80.4)

[a] Characteristics are listed for subjects who completed the study.

Table 2
Total body weight loss across aspiration therapy trials

Study Group	Week 26 (Percent Total Body Weight Loss)	Week 52 (Percent Total Body Weight Loss)	Week 104 (Percent Total Body Weight Loss)
Mexico pilot study[13] N = 9	9.7 ± 5.7	15.9 ± 8.3 (n = 6)	—
US pilot study control group N = 4	3.7 ± 4.3	5.9 ± 5.0	—
US pilot study aspiration therapy group N = 10	14.8 ± 3.9	18.6 ± 2.3	21.2 ± 2.8 (n = 7)
Sweden pilot study N = 22	14.8 ± 6.3	—	—
PATHWAY control group N = 60	2.8 ± 4.6	3.5 ± 6.0	—
PATHWAY aspiration therapy group N = 111	9.1 ± 6.1	12.1 ± 9.6	—
European superobesity pilot study N = 11	14.5	21.4	25.5 (n = 6)

Cardiometabolic Risk Factors

In the PATHWAY, systolic and diastolic blood pressure decreased and fasting plasma lipids improved across the study groups but no significant difference in improvement was detected between subjects in the aspiration therapy group and the control group. Significantly more subjects in the aspiration therapy group, however, discontinued all antihypertensive medications compared with subjects in the control group (62% and 10% respectively, $P<.0001$). Additionally, more subjects in the aspiration therapy group discontinued all lipid-lowering medications compared with subjects in the control group (23% and 8% respectively, $P = .593$). In the Swedish pilot study, there was a significant reduction in C-reactive protein as well as a trend toward reductions in fasting plasma glucose concentrations and hemoglobin A_{1c}. Moreover, in the 7 subjects with diabetes at the start of the trial, fasting glucose decreased from 9.4 mmol/L to 7.4 mmol/L ($P = .04$), and 3 subjects decreased or completely stopped all antidiabetic medications at 6 months. These improvements in cardiometabolic risk factors are expected for the amount of weight loss seen in these trials and likely due to the weight loss and not an independent effect of aspiration therapy.

Although plasma alanine aminotransferase (ALT) concentration is not typically considered a cardiometabolic risk factor, plasma ALT concentrations correlate with all-cause mortality,[18] risk of developing diabetes,[19] and nonalcoholic fatty liver disease.[20] A significant decrease in plasma ALT concentrations was seen the US pilot study in the aspiration therapy group after 52 weeks of therapy (20.6 ± 2.6 IU/L and 12.8 ± 1.9 IU/L; $P = .014$). A trend in a decrease in plasma ALT concentration was seen in both the Mexico pilot study at 26 weeks (55.7 ± 55.2 IU/L and 21.6 ± 6.0 IU/L; $P = .076$) and the Swedish pilot study (0.56 ± 0.34 microkatal [μkat]/L and 0.45 ± 0.31 μkat/L; $P = .080$). As with the cardiometabolic risk factors, the changes in ALT seen in these trials are expected with the weight loss achieved in these trials and likely not an independent effect of aspiration therapy.

Eating Behaviors

Subjects with a history of an eating disorder were excluded from these trials. In both the US pilot study and PATHWAY, subjects were additionally screened with the Eating Disorder Examination Questionnaire[11] and the Questionnaire on Eating and Weight Patterns Revised.[21] Subjects in these trials repeated these evaluations again at 12 weeks or 14 weeks, 24 weeks or 28 weeks, and 52 weeks. One subject in control arm of the PATHWAY had evidence of binge eating disorder at 28 weeks. None of the subjects treated with aspiration therapy in either US study developed bulimia or binge eating disorder.

Subjects in the US pilot study also underwent serial evaluations for depression with the Beck Depression Inventory-II,[22] eating behavioral traits with the Three-Factor Eating Questionnaire,[10] and hunger with hunger visual analog scales.[23] One subject in the control group had evidence of depression at week 24, but no change in the Beck Depression Inventory-II was detected in the aspiration therapy group. The aspiration therapy group showed improvement in all 3 measures of the Three-Factor Eating Questionnaire, including improved restraint, less disinhibition, and decreased hunger. Moreover, despite aspirating one-third of calories after a meal, there were no significant changes in visual analog scales for hunger, increased thoughts of food, increased cravings, or decreased feelings of fullness in aspiration therapy group subjects.[14] Lastly, number of aspiration sessions per day were measured by determining the number of times the connectors were used to open the skin port in the PATHWAY. Subjects averaged 2.5 connections for aspiration per day for the first 14 weeks of therapy and 2 connections for aspiration per day for the remainder of the trial. No subjects were connecting for aspiration more than 3 times per day on average.

Taken together, these data demonstrate that aspiration therapy does not induce binge eating disorder or bulimia. Additionally, they suggest that aspiration of calories after food has been delivered to the stomach may result in neurohormonal signals that relay information about calorie ingestion to the brain before the calories are removed with aspiration. This may explain the lack of hunger experienced by patients performing aspiration therapy even after removing up to a third of the calories consumed.

Psychological Evaluations

Quality of life was measured with the Impact of Weight on Quality of Life (IWQOL)[24] score in the PATHWAY, with increases in all 5 measures of quality of life (physical function, self-esteem, sexual life, public distress, and work) in both the aspiration therapy and control groups but significantly greater increases in the total IWQOL score in the aspiration therapy group compared with the control group ($P = .03$). The 36-Item Short Form Survey quality-of-life questionnaire[25] was used in Mexico pilot study, with a small decrease in emotional well-being and pain scores at 26 weeks compared with baseline but no changes 52 weeks compared with baseline in the 6 subjects who completed 52 weeks of therapy. These findings were likely related to pain from the original A-Tube design, which led to changes in design to the current smooth all-silicone A-Tube. Moreover, these 6 subjects had a small improvement in physical function at week 52 compared with baseline (91.7 ± 11.7 and 79.2 ± 8.6, respectively; $P<.05$). The EuroQol (EQ) EQ-5[26] and EQ visual analog scale[27] were used in the Swedish pilot study and demonstrated improvements of 0.73 to 0.83 ($P = .015$) and 61 ± 15 to 73 ± 19 ($P = .003$) from baseline to 26 weeks. Taken together, these data suggest that with the current AspireAssist System, aspiration therapy leads to an improved quality of life.

COMPLICATIONS

Most of the study-related adverse events across aspiration therapy trials are consistent with known complications from PEG tubes[4] and no deaths have been reported. In the largest study, the PATHWAY, 5 SAEs (3.6%) occurred during the 52-week study, including[5,16]

- One subject with perioperative pain requiring 2 separate overnight stays in the hospital with pain medications, each counted separately as SAEs
- One case of mild perioperative peritonitis treated with 2-night hospital stay and intravenous antibiotics
- One postprocedure mild ulceration treated with A-Tube removal
- One case of A-Tube fungal colonization treated with A-Tube

Additionally, 1 SAE was recorded after the 52-week study during the optional continuation period, which consisted of a fistula tract that developed superior to the A-Tube tract. This was successfully treated with A-Tube removal. No SAEs were reported in a US pilot trial,[14] European pilot trial,[15] or European superobesity pilot trial.[17] One SAE occurred in the pilot trial in Mexico: a subject who had been noncompliant with the study protocol had a migration of the intragastric bumper into the A-Tube fistula tract, likely related to external traction the subject had placed on the tube. The

A-tube was removed surgically and was not replaced. Other nonserious adverse events, which required surgery or hospitalization, include

- Mexico pilot study
  - One patient admitted overnight for pain control after A-Tube placement
  - Two subjects required surgical fistula tract closure due to persistent fistula 17 to 28 days after the A-Tube was removed. No attempt was made at endoscopic closure of the fistula tract due to the lack of equipment and endoscopic expertise at the Mexico study site.
- US pilot study: none
- Swedish pilot study:
  - One patient admitted overnight for pain control after A-Tube placement
  - One patient hospitalized for drainage of an aseptic intra-abdominal fluid collection 10 days after A-Tube placement
- PATHWAY: only hospitalizations listed in SAE section
- European superobesity study: none

The most common nonserious adverse events across the studies include abdominal pain after A-Tube placement, granulation tissue, intermittent abdominal discomfort, and peristomal irritation or bleeding. **Table 3** lists all adverse events for the PATHWAY, which contains data on the largest number of patients. Most of the adverse events were rated mild or moderate and resolved spontaneously or with standard medical therapy within 7 days of occurrence.[5]

Table 3
PATHWAY trial nonserious adverse events

Event Description	Subjects (%)
Peristomal granulation tissue	45 (40.5)
Abdominal pain ≤4 wk after A-Tube placement	42 (37.8)
Intermittent abdominal discomfort	18 (16.2)
Nausea/vomiting	20 (18.0)
Peristomal irritation	19 (17.1)
Possible or confirmed bacterial infection	15 (13.5)
Abdominal pain >4 wk after A-Tube placement	9 (8.1)
Dyspepsia (composite: acid reflux, heart burn, hiccups, belching)	7 (6.3)
Peristomal inflammation	6 (5.4)
Peristomal discharge	5 (4.5)
Change in bowel habits (constipation or diarrhea)	5 (4.5)
Hypokalemia	4 (3.6)
Accidental A-Tube dislodgement or trauma	3 (2.7)
Peristomal bleeding	2 (1.8)
Peristomal fungal infection	2 (1.8)
Other miscellaneous single events (A-Tube replacement, broken tooth veneer, buried bumper, ecchymosis, fever, free air in abdomen after A-Tube placement, peristomal ulceration, persistent fistula, worsening bilateral leg edema, hand pain, substernal discomfort, peritonitis, stomach spasm)	13 (0.9) each

ELECTROLYTES

Removal of gastric acid can result in hypokalemia. In both the Mexico pilot study and US pilot study, subjects took daily omeprazole and potassium supplementation to prevent hypokalemia. In the other studies, omeprazole and potassium supplementation were only used if patients had evidence of hypokalemia. A total of 6 subjects developed hypokalemia with serum potassium concentrations between 3.2 mEq/L and 3.7 mEq/L in all the studies. These subjects were all managed successfully with potassium supplementation.

MECHANISMS OF ACTION FOR WEIGHT LOSS

The most obvious mechanism for weight loss with aspiration therapy is the removal of a portion of calories consumed before absorption in the gastrointestinal tract. Evaluation of the efficiency of aspiration revealed the effect of the timing and amount of food consumed on percent of calories aspirated. Aspirating 20 minutes after a 450-kcal meal was ingested resulted in removal of approximately 30% of the calories consumed whereas aspirating 60 minutes after the meal was ingested resulted in removal of only 17% of the calories consumed. In contrast, aspirating at 20 minutes or 60 minutes after a large (800-kcal meal) resulted in equivalent removal of calories consumed, approximately 28% and 27%, respectively.[14]

What is less obvious is that aspiration of calories did not account for all of the weight loss achieved in subjects in the US pilot study. For these subjects, only 80% of the weight seen was due to aspiration even when estimating that 30% of all calories were aspirated. Given that patients did not aspirate snacks, frequently aspirated only 2 times per day, and did not always aspirate 20 minutes after a meal, the weight loss attributed to aspiration of calories alone is likely significantly less than 80%.[14] Therefore, more than 20% of the weight loss seen with aspiration therapy is likely due to a reduction in food intake. Moreover, 78% of subjects in the PATHWAY randomized controlled trial of aspiration therapy reported either significantly or somewhat decreased calorie consumption.[16] There are multiple factors that may explain a reduction in calorie intake:

- Food particles must be less than or equal to 5 mm to reliably fit through the A-Tube.
  - Patients are required to chew food significantly longer to reach optimal particle size.
  - This results in cessation of meals with fewer calories consumed
- Gastric contents must contain enough liquid to flow out of the A-Tube.
  - Patients increase water consumption with meals to facilitate aspiration.
  - This enhances sense of satiation without additional calories
- The fistula between the gastric wall and abdominal wall may affect gastric accommodation during a meal.
  - Patients report early satiation with a meal after A-Tube implantation but before the Skin-Port is placed for aspiration after meals.
- Gastric aspirate can be seen through the clear patient and drain lines.
  - Patients report that healthy, lower-calorie food choices have a normal appearance on aspiration.
  - Less healthy food choices, for example, fried food, have an unappealing appearance on aspiration and lead to a reduction in consumption of those foods.

In addition, compensatory eating or sensation of hunger did not occur in subjects after aspiration in either the US pilot trial or the PATHWAY randomized controlled trials, as discussed previously.[14,16] Assuming that these subjects had normal physiologic controls for satiation and satiety, it is possible that allowing calories to enter into the stomach resulted in neurohormonal signals from the gut to the brain, indicating a larger meal was consumed than was ultimately absorbed. None of the studies performed with aspiration therapy, however, has been designed to determine the physiologic effects of aspiration therapy on gut hormones involved in appetite regulation. Further research in this area is needed.

SUMMARY

Aspiration therapy performed with the recently FDA-approved AspireAssist System results in significant weight loss across studies both in and outside the United States, with approximately 3 times more weight loss seen in patients undergoing aspiration therapy in conjunction with lifestyle therapy compared with subjects undergoing lifestyle therapy alone. Markers of cardiometabolic health and plasma ALT improved with aspiration therapy, but this is expected for the amount of weight loss achieved with aspiration therapy and not likely an independent effect. Quality of life also improved, despite implantation of a device that is partially outside the body on the skin surface. SAEs were low or did not occur in the trials completed to date and most nonserious adverse events resolved spontaneously or with standard medical therapy within 7 days. Electrolyte abnormalities, namely hypokalemia, were uncommon, with only 6 patients developing mild hypokalemia, which was treated successfully with potassium supplementation.

Although the obvious cause of weight loss is the removal of up to 30% of calories with a meal, other mechanisms also contribute to the weight loss achieved with aspiration therapy. Patients eat less food at meals due to the mealtime behaviors that are required to aspirate gastric contents, namely chewing food into very small food particles and drinking enough water during the meal to allow flow out of the A-Tube. In addition, the A-Tube may alter the stomach's ability to accommodate food during a meal because subjects self-reported early satiety with meals before skin port conversion and initiation of aspiration after meals. Patients also made healthy food choices to avoid unpleasant-appearing gastric aspirate of unhealthy food choices. Lastly, aspiration of calories does not result in increased hunger or compensatory eating, which suggests that the mechanisms that signal satiation with a meal are still activated despite up to 30% of those calorie removed.

Further research is needed to better understand the mechanisms involved in weight loss with aspiration therapy and to identify patients who are most likely to benefit from this therapy. Moreover, additional research in patients with a BMI greater than 55 kg/m^2 is also needed to determine the risks and benefits in this difficult-to-treat population. Despite these additional research questions, the evidence available confirms that aspiration therapy provides a safe and effective method for weight loss in patients with a BMI between 35 kg/m^2 and 55 kg/m^2 who have not been successful with lifestyle therapy alone.

REFERENCES

1. Hussain SS, Bloom SR. The regulation of food intake by the gut-brain axis: implications for obesity. Int J Obes 2013;37:625–33.
2. French SA, Epstein LH, Jeffery RW, et al. Eating behavior dimensions. Associations with energy intake and body weight. A review. Appetite 2012;59:541–9.
3. The Look ARG. Eight-year weight losses with an intensive lifestyle intervention: the look AHEAD study. Obesity (Silver Spring) 2014;22:5–13.

4. Rahnemai-Azar AA, Rahnemaiazar AA, Naghshizadian R, et al. Percutaneous endoscopic gastrostomy: Indications, technique, complications and management. World J Gastroenterol 2014;20:7739–51.
5. FDA. Summary of safety and effectiveness data (SSED) AspireAssist. In: FDA, editor. 2016. p. 1–36.
6. Sullivan S, Kumar N, Edmundowicz SA, et al. ASGE position statement on endoscopic bariatric therapies in clinical practice. Gastrointest Endosc 2015;82:767–72.
7. American Psychiatric Association, DSM-5 Task Force. Diagnostic and statistical manual of mental disorders: DSM-5. Washington, DC: American Psychiatric Association; 2013.
8. Parker K, Brennan L. Measurement of disordered eating in bariatric surgery candidates: a systematic review of the literature. Obes Res Clin Pract 2015;9:12–25.
9. Yanovski SZ, Marcus MD, Wadden TA, et al. The questionnaire on eating and weight patterns-5 (QEWP-5): an updated screening instrument for binge eating disorder. Int J Eat Disord 2015;48:259–61.
10. Stunkard AJ, Messick S. The three-factor eating questionnaire to measure dietary restraint, disinhibition and hunger. J Psychosom Res 1985;29:71–83.
11. Fairburn CG. Cognitive behavior therapy and eating disorders. New York: Guildford Press; 2008.
12. Gormally J, Black S, Daston S, et al. The assessment of binge eating severity among obese persons. Addict Behav 1982;7:47–55.
13. Sullivan S, Cruz P, Lavalle Gonzales F. Single-arm pilot study for safety and efficacy of aspiration therapy in Mexico. In press.
14. Sullivan S, Stein R, Jonnalagadda S, et al. Aspiration therapy leads to weight loss in obese subjects: a pilot study. Gastroenterology 2013;145:1245–52.e1–5.
15. Forssell H, Noren E. A novel endoscopic weight loss therapy using gastric aspiration: results after 6 months. Endoscopy 2015;47:68–71.
16. Thompson CC, Dayyeh BKA, Kushner R, et al. 381 the AspireAssist is an effective tool in the treatment of class II and class III obesity: results of a one-year clinical trial. Gastroenterology 2016;150:S86.
17. Machytka E, Turro R, Huberty V, et al. Mo1944 aspiration therapy in super obese patients - pilot trial. Gastroenterology 2016;150:S822–3.
18. Kunutsor SK, Apekey TA, Seddoh D, et al. Liver enzymes and risk of all-cause mortality in general populations: a systematic review and meta-analysis. Int J Epidemiol 2014;43:187–201.
19. Fraser A, Harris R, Sattar N, et al. Alanine aminotransferase, γ-glutamyltransferase, and incident diabetes: the British Women's Heart and Health Study and meta-analysis. Diabetes Care 2009;32:741–50.
20. Browning JD, Szczepaniak LS, Dobbins R, et al. Prevalence of hepatic steatosis in an urban population in the United States: Impact of ethnicity. Hepatology 2004;40:1387–95.
21. ZelitchYanovski S. Binge eating disorder: current knowledge and future directions. Obes Res 1993;1:306–24.
22. Beck A, Steer R, Brown G. Manual for the beck depression inventory. San Antonio (TX): The Psychological Corporation; 1996.
23. Flint A, Raben A, Blundell JE, et al. Reproducibility, power and validity of visual analogue scales in assessment of appetite sensations in single test meal studies. Int J Obes Relat Metab Disord 2000;24:38–48.
24. Kolotkin RL, Crosby RD, Kosloski KD, et al. Development of a brief measure to assess quality of life in obesity. Obes Res 2001;9:102–11.

25. Corica F, Corsonello A, Apolone G, et al. Construct validity of the short form-36 health survey and its relationship with BMI in obese outpatients. Obesity (Silver Spring) 2006;14:1429–37.
26. Krabbe PFM, Stouthard MEA, Essink-Bot M-L, et al. The effect of adding a cognitive dimension to the euroqol multiattribute health-status classification system. J Clin Epidemiol 1999;52:293–301.
27. Parkin D, Rice N, Jacoby A, et al. Use of a visual analogue scale in a daily patient diary: modelling cross-sectional time-series data on health-related quality of life. Soc Sci Med 2004;59:351–60.

Small Bowel Target Devices and Techniques

Steven A. Edmundowicz, MD

KEYWORDS

- Obesity • Endoscopy • Endoscopic bariatric therapies
- Small bowel endoscopic interventions • Endoscopic sleeve

KEY POINTS

- The small bowel is important in the management of obesity, type 2 diabetes mellitus, and metabolic syndrome. Bariatric surgical therapies have focused on the small bowel for decades.
- New understanding of the mechanisms of obesity and type 2 diabetes mellitus as they relate to the small bowel have led to the development of endoscopic bariatric therapies that focus in this region.
- Endoluminal sleeves function by bypassing the proximal duodenum and have been shown to be effective in the short-term management of obesity and diabetes.
- Dual-path enteral bypass functions by delivering enteral contents rapidly to the ileum and represents a new treatment of both obesity and diabetes.

INTRODUCTION

The small bowel plays a significant role in weight management and management of type 2 diabetes mellitus (T2DM). Manipulation of the small bowel has been used in surgical weight loss procedures for decades and was initially established by creating malabsorption to facilitate weight loss.[1,2] Further work has identified other mechanisms of action that are becoming key to understanding the role of the small bowel in obesity and T2DM.[3,4] Key clinical observations in patients who had gastric bypass showed that weight loss and reversal of diabetes can occur and are largely caused by the bypass of the proximal small bowel. Recent reviews of the physiology of small bowel manipulation have identified several possible mechanisms of action for small bowel devices that lead to weight loss and control of T2DM.[5–7] Two main mechanisms of action for procedures and surgeries of the small bowel to affect obesity and T2DM

Disclosure: Discloses contracted research for ReShape Medical, GI Dynamics, Aspire Bariatrics, USGI Medical, Obalon Therapeutics; consultant and stockholder in Elira and Endostim; consultant and medical advisor for Olympus, Boston Scientific, and Medtronic.
Digestive Health Center, University of Colorado Hospital, University of Colorado School of Medicine, Mail Stop F735, Anschutz Outpatient Pavilion, 1635 Aurora Court, Aurora, CO 80045, USA
E-mail address: steven.edmundowicz@ucdenver.edu

are foregut exclusion and rapid delivery of food to the ileum. Both have been implicated in invoking an incretin pathway for improvement in obesity and resolution of T2DM but understanding of these mechanisms is far from complete.[8] These concepts and the surgical therapies are expanded on elsewhere (see Zubaidah Nor Hanipah and Philip R Schauer's article, "Surgical Treatment of Obesity and Diabetes"; and Lee M. Kaplan's article, "What Bariatric Surgery Can Teach Us About Endoluminal Treatment of Obesity and Metabolic Disorders," in this issue). Endoscopic bariatric therapies that target the small bowel and have been used in humans include endoluminal sleeves, duodenal mucosal resurfacing, and partial stream intestinal bypass procedures. Duodenal mucosal resurfacing are the focus of a following article in this series (see Alan D. Cherrington and colleagues' article, "Hydrothermal Duodenal Mucosal Resurfacing: Role in the Treatment of Metabolic Disease," in this issue). The remaining 2 approaches have been used both in animal studies[9,10] and in humans and have been found to be effective in the treatment of obesity and T2DM.

ENDOLUMINAL SLEEVES
Duodenal Jejunal Bypass Liner

In an attempt to mimic the small bowel bypass of the Roux-en-Y gastric bypass procedures without surgery, Rodriquez-Grunert and colleagues[11] described an endoluminal sleeve device that could be deployed endoscopically with anchors in the duodenum that essentially provided a lumen within the lumen of the proximal small bowel, prohibiting contact between the mucosa and ingested contents. The sleeve also did not allow bile and pancreatic secretions to contact the food stream until the end of the sleeve some 60 cm downstream from the major papilla. The resulting bypass of proximal small bowel mucosa had a profound effect on glucose metabolism and led to weight loss and improvement of T2DM. This device was brought to further human trials and marketed outside the United States as the EndoBarrier (GI Dynamics, Lexington MA).[12,13] The system consists of a 60-cm Teflon polymer sleeve, a nitinol crown anchoring system at the proximal end with barbs that penetrate the duodenal wall, and is designed to be deployed in the duodenal bulb (**Fig. 1**A). The sleeve is encapsulated in a delivery system that is introduced over a guidewire into the duodenum. The EndoBarrier is deployed with endoscopic and fluoroscopic guidance to direct placement of the anchoring system into the duodenal bulb and allow the deployed sleeve to cover the proximal small bowel (**Fig. 1**B). While the device is in place, contents from the stomach pass through the lumen of the sleeve and are

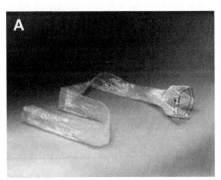
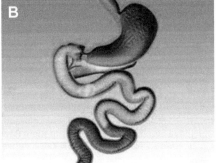

Fig. 1. (A) The EndoBarrier with nitinol crown and Teflon sleeve. (B) The EndoBarrier in place. (*Courtesy of* GI Dynamics Inc, Lexington, MA.)

delivered into the proximal small bowel without contact with the mucosa or digestive enzymes from the biliary tree or pancreas. The sleeves were left in place for varying time intervals (3–12 months) and then removed endoscopically with a retrieval device that collapses the nitinol anchor into an endoscopic hood to protect the gastrointestinal (GI) tract as it is withdrawn. The early clinical experience with the device in open-label trials has been encouraging, with excess weight loss (EWL) in the 25% to 35% range when the sleeve is left in place longer than 3 months.[13–15] Investigators also noticed a prompt and significant improvement in hemoglobin A1c (HbA1c) levels. This finding led to additional studies, including randomized controlled trials, which typically result in less weight loss than open-label studies. The results of the reported trials were reviewed in a meta-analysis by Abu Dayyeh and colleagues[16] in 2015. This meta-analysis showed that, in the open label studies, more than 25% EWL was achieved with the device. Three studies enrolling 105 patients achieved an EWL of 35.3% (95% confidence interval [CI], 24.6–46.1) at 12 months.[13–15] Four randomized controlled trials compared 12 to 24 weeks of treatment with the EndoBarrier duodenal jejunal bypass liner (90 subjects) with a sham or control arm (84 subjects).[12,14,17,18] The mean EWL difference compared with a control group was significant at 9.4% (95% CI, 8.26–10.65). Even with short-term (3-month) use the glycosylated hemoglobin was significantly improved compared with controls.[19] Patient tolerance of the device has been variable and early removal is necessary for symptoms in a percentage of patients. Complications related to the sleeve were reported in all the trials. The cumulative complication rate for the clinical trials analyzed in the meta-analysis included 271 implanted patients and reported serious adverse events, including sleeve migration (4.9%), GI bleeding (3.86%), sleeve obstruction (3.4%), liver abscess (0.126%), cholangitis (0.126%), acute cholecystitis (0.126%), and esophageal perforation (0.126%) (secondary to trauma from an uncovered barb at withdrawal).[16]

Although the device has been used widely outside the United States, it has not been approved to be marketed for clinical use in the United States by the US Food and Drug Administration (FDA). A pivotal multicenter randomized controlled trial was initiated in the United States in 2013. However, this 21-center trial had enrollment suspended in March 2015 because of a safety issue with an increased incidence of hepatic abscesses being reported. According to a press release on the GI Dynamics Web site,[20] the trial was placed on hold when 4 cases of hepatic abscess were noted in the 325 randomized subjects. Negotiations with the FDA on a mitigation plan stalled and the trial has not been restarted as of the date of submission of this article. Results from the incompletely enrolled trial are difficult to interpret and have been presented in abstract form.[21]

The device is still being sold and used outside the United States with reported good results. A recent report describes improvement in liver function in subjects with nonalcoholic fatty liver disease treated with the EndoBarrier.[22] A single center also reported its site experience with the device, identifying the side effects seen with clinical use of the EndoBarrier.[23] Eighty percent of patients designated to receive the device were able to complete the prescribed therapy without premature removal or a complication.[23,24] The same center recently reported its patients' experience 12 months after the EndoBarrier had been removed.[25] Fifty-nine patients completed the 12-month follow-up after explantation. During this period, body weight increased by 5.6 kg (standard deviation [SD], 6.4 kg) (P<.001) and HbA1c level increased from 65 mmol/mol (SD, 17 mmol/mol) to 70 mmol/mol (SD, 20 mmol/mol) (P<.001). Body weight remained 8.0 kg (SD, 8.6 kg) (P<.001) lower than before implantation; that is, corresponding with a net total body weight loss of 7.4% (SD, 7.6%) (P<.001) (**Fig. 2**). The investigators call for a change in strategy to maintain the benefits of the EndoBarrier in their patients.[25]

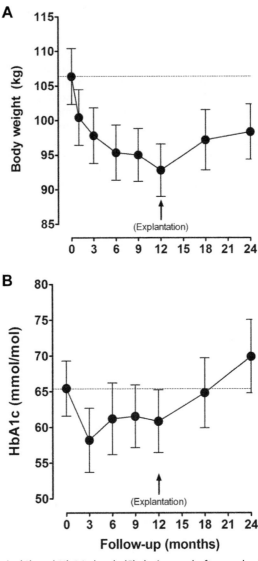

Fig. 2. Weight regain (*A*) and HbA1c levels (*B*) during and after explantation of the Endo-Barrier device in 59 patients. (*From* Betzel B, Koehestanie P, Homan J, et al. Changes in glycemic control and body weight after explantation of the duodenal-jejunal bypass liner. Gastrointest Endosc 2017;85(2):409–15.)

The EndoBarrier has created much excitement with its arrival in the bariatric space and it has led to increased investment and research in endoscopic bariatric therapies that have moved the field forward. The obstacles before it now include mitigation of severe complications (hepatic abscesses) and demonstration of a strategy to maintain the positive effects of the device long term. It is our hope that these hurdles are not insurmountable and that beneficial effects of this technology can be preserved.

Gastroduodenojejunal Bypass Sleeve

A second concept in small bowel bypass sleeves is the gastroduodenojejunal sleeve (ValenTx, Inc, Maple Grove, MN). This 120-cm fluoropolymer sleeve is implanted with endoscopic techniques and then secured in place with a laparoscopic procedure to expose the gastroesophageal junction (GEJ) and guide the placement of transmural suture anchors.[26] The implanted sleeve extends from the GEJ to the jejunum. All oral intake is diverted through the sleeve and delivered to the jejunum without contacting the proximal small bowel mucosa or mixing with pancreatic and biliary secretions until that junction. Clinical trials have been conducted in morbidly obese patients. The patients underwent endoscopic and laparoscopic sleeve placement and were then maintained on a liquid diet for 2 weeks followed by a pureed diet for 2 weeks, then a regular diet. A total of 37 patients (mean body mass index [BMI], 42 kg/m^2) are described in 2 reports in the literature.[26,27] The first group of patients studied had the sleeve implanted for 12 weeks.[26] Of the 24 patients enrolled, 2 were not implanted and 5 had early explantation for symptoms of pain or dysphagia. The symptoms resolved once the sleeves were removed. One subject had the sleeve endoscopically manipulated to remove a kink in the stomach that limited food passage 4 weeks after placement. The 17 subjects who completed 12 weeks of therapy had 39.7% EWL.[27] The patients reported early satiety and reduced food intake during the study period. All devices were removed endoscopically using endoscopic scissors or ablation catheters to remove the anchoring sutures. The sleeves were then withdrawn through the mouth.

Thirteen subjects were enrolled in a second trial using the same sleeve, which was implanted for a total of 12 months.[27] One subject could not be implanted and 2 subjects required early sleeve explantation because of symptoms. Ten subjects kept the sleeves in place for 12 months. Six of the subjects had functional sleeves in place with complete attachment of the esophageal cuff at the end of the 12-month period. These subjects lost a total of 54% EWL. The other 4 subjects had partially detached sleeves and lower EWL. Eleven subjects in the 2 trials had T2DM and all improved with therapy (stopped medications or showed improvement in glycosylated hemoglobin). This preliminary experience suggests that the gastroduodenojejunal sleeve is a potentially viable device for significant weight loss and improvement in T2DM. Resolution of the anchoring issues and device evolution to a completely endoluminally delivered device seems essential for this particular design to be successful.

DUAL-PATH ENTERAL BYPASS

A novel approach for the treatment of obesity and T2DM is the endoscopic creation of an intestinal bypass. Ryou and colleagues[28] developed a system to create an enteroentero bypass using self-assembling rare earth magnets (incisionless magnetic anastomosis system [IMAS], GI Windows, Stoughton, MA). The advantages of magnetic anastomosis creation in the setting of obesity therapy are significant. The anastomosis can be created slowly (over days) with tissue ischemia. The anastomosis is noninflammatory after formation, therefore it does not seem to need to be maintained with stents or other devices. The entire process is done endoluminally so there is no adhesion formation. This approach has been studied in the porcine model[10] and applied to humans in a pilot study.[29] The concept in humans was to create a dual-lumen proximal jejunal to distal ileal anastomosis that allows partially digested contents to pass rapidly to the distal ileum (**Fig. 3**). Unlike the established surgical jejunoileal bypass procedure this endoluminal therapy creates a partial

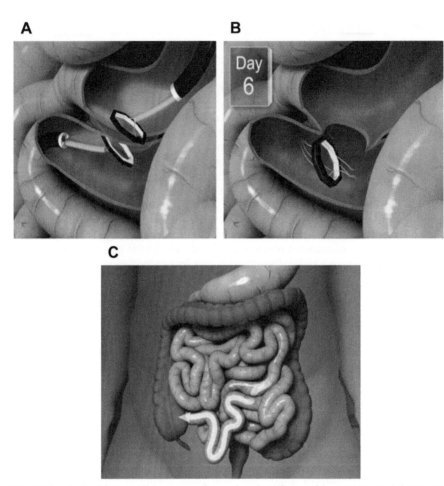

Fig. 3. The dual-path enteral bypass performed with self-assembling magnets. (*A*) Two endoscopists perform upper and lower endoscopy to the regions of the proximal jejunum and ileum. Once the endoscopes are in approximation, the self-assembling magnet catheters are passed into the lumen and the octagonal magnets form. The magnets are moved into position and they couple with no intervening structures. The magnets are then released and the endoscopes removed. (*B*) Approximately 6 days later, the pressure ischemia creates a communication between the two lumens and the magnets pass into the intestine and out of the body. (*C*) The dual-lumen nature of the enteroentero bypass allowing enteral contents to flow to all areas of the small bowel and eventually to the colon. (*Courtesy of* GI Windows, Waltham, MA.)

bypass (dual pathway) allowing partially digested food and digestive enzyme exposure to the mucosa of the entire small bowel.

The pilot human trial with this technique was presented at Digestive Disease Week 2016.[29] Ten morbidly obese subjects (mean BMI, 41 kg/m^2) underwent an enteroenteral bypass with the IMAS under laparoscopic observation to ensure adequate anastomosis formation. The self-assembling magnets were positioned by 2 endoscopists, one performing an enteroscopy (proximal jejunum) and a second performing a simultaneous retrograde ileoscopy with a colonoscope to a region in the ileum upstream from the ileocecal valve. The magnets were then passed through the operating channels of the endoscopes and allowed to couple with no intervening structures. The octagonal magnets were then released to develop the compression anastomosis over several days. All subjects were placed on a liquid diet initially and advanced to soft diet for 2 weeks, but following this no specific dietary direction was provided. Subjects had a barium upper GI radiograph study at 2 weeks to confirm anastomotic patency and endoscopy at 2 and 6 months to visualize the anastomosis.

Weight loss at 6 months was seen in all subjects, with 10.6% total weight loss (28.3% EWL). Three prediabetic and 4 diabetic patients (T2DM) all improved significantly, with normalization of glycosylated hemoglobin levels. No serious adverse events were encountered. Diarrhea persisted in several patients and was managed symptomatically with diet and or medications.

This pilot study presents a promising development in endoscopic bariatric therapy. Although requiring a dual endoscopy, the IMAS resulted in a widely patent anastomosis that does not have a residual foreign body that would require removal or maintenance. This outcome suggests that this procedure will be long lasting and not require repeat procedures or modifications to maintain its effect. Although larger and longer term studies are needed to confirm the findings of this preliminary report, the potential for this treatment to have a major role in the endoscopic therapy for obesity and T2DM is significant and very encouraging.

DUODENAL MUCOSAL RESURFACING

Duodenal mucosal resurfacing (DMR) involves hydrothermal ablation of the duodenal mucosa using the Revita DMR (Fractyl, Waltham, MA).[30] The procedure is performed by advancing a catheter into the duodenum that can inject saline for circumferential submucosal lift distal to the ampulla of Vater, followed by inflation and circulation of heated water in a balloon on the catheter for circumferential ablation of the mucosa under direct visualization. This therapy is not associated with significant weight loss, but improves glycemic control in T2DM.[30] Early experience with DMR has been postulated to have a significant effect on the neuroendocrine cells of the epithelium, leading to an improvement in T2DM and prediabetic states. The Revita DMR procedure is discussed in detail elsewhere (see Alan D. Cherrington and colleagues' article, "Hydrothermal Duodenal Mucosal Resurfacing: Role in the Treatment of Metabolic Disease," in this issue).

SUMMARY

The small bowel has become a favored target for endoscopic therapies to provide treatment of morbid obesity, T2DM, and the metabolic syndromes. Adaptation and evolution of the techniques discussed earlier are already in progress and are likely to lead to new techniques and treatments for these conditions. Resolving the anchoring issue with sleeve technology, improving duodenal resurfacing, and developing internal anastomotic systems that are easier to use will provide new approaches to endoscopic therapy for obesity and metabolic disorders that will revolutionize this space. In addition, the development of a durable therapy for these conditions that does not need to be maintained or repeated will push endoscopic bariatric therapies into a new era in the management of these conditions.

REFERENCES

1. Buchwald H, Avidor Y, Braunwald E, et al. Bariatric surgery: a systematic review and meta-analysis. JAMA 2004;292:1724–37.

2. Schauer PR, Burguera B, Ikramuddin S, et al. Effect of laparoscopic Roux-en Y gastric bypass on type 2 diabetes mellitus. Ann Surg 2003;238:467–84 [discussion: 84–5].

3. Cohen R, le Roux CW, Papamargaritis D, et al. Role of proximal gut exclusion from food on glucose homeostasis in patients with type 2 diabetes. Diabet Med 2013;30:1482–6.

4. Melvin A, le Roux CW, Docherty NG. The gut as an endocrine organ: role in the regulation of food intake and body weight. Curr Atheroscler Rep 2016;18:49.

5. Duca FA, Bauer PV, Hamr SC, et al. Glucoregulatory relevance of small intestinal nutrient sensing in physiology, bariatric surgery, and pharmacology. Cell Metab 2015;22:367–80.

6. Theodorakis MJ, Carlson O, Michopoulos S, et al. Human duodenal enteroendocrine cells: source of both incretin peptides, GLP-1 and GIP. Am J Physiol Endocrinol Metab 2006;290:E550–9.

7. Rubino F, Forgione A, Cummings DE, et al. The mechanism of diabetes control after gastrointestinal bypass surgery reveals a role of the proximal small intestine in the pathophysiology of type 2 diabetes. Ann Surg 2006;244:741–9.

8. Bose M, Oliván B, Teixeira J, et al. Do incretins play a role in the remission of type 2 diabetes after gastric bypass surgery: what are the evidence? Obes Surg 2009; 19:217–29.

9. Muñoz R, Carmody JS, Stylopoulos N, et al. Isolated duodenal exclusion increases energy expenditure and improves glucose homeostasis in diet-induced obese rats. Am J Physiol Regul Integr Comp Physiol 2012;303(10): R985–93.

10. Ryou M, Agoston AT, Thompson CC. Endoscopic intestinal bypass creation by using self-assembling magnets in a porcine model. Gastrointest Endosc 2015; 2016(83):821–5.

11. Rodriguez-Grunert L, GalvaoNeto MP, Alamo M, et al. First human experience with endoscopically delivered and retrieved duodenal jejunal bypass sleeve. Surg Obes Relat Dis 2008;4:55–9.

12. Gersin KS, Rothstein RI, Rosenthal RJ, et al. Sham-controlled trial of an endoscopic duodenojejunal bypass liner for preoperative weight loss in bariatric surgery candidates. Gastrointest Endosc 2010;71:976–82.

13. de Moura EG, Martins BC, Lopes GS, et al. Metabolic improvements in obese type 2 diabetes subjects implanted for 1 year with an endoscopically deployed duodenal-jejunal bypass liner. Diabetes Technol Ther 2012;14:183–9.

14. Koehestanie P, de Jonge C, Berends FJ, et al. The effect of the endoscopic duodenal- bypass liner on obesity and type 2 diabetes mellitus, a multicenter randomized controlled trial. Ann Surg 2014;260:984–92.

15. Munoz R, Dominguez A, Munoz F, et al. Baseline glycated hemoglobin levels are associated with duodenal-jejunal bypass liner induced weight loss in obese patients. Surg Endosc 2014;28:1056–62.

16. Abu Dayyeh BK, Kumar N, Edmundowicz SA, et al. ASGE Bariatric Endoscopy Task Force systematic review and meta-analysis assessing the ASGE PIVI thresholds for adopting endoscopic bariatric therapies. Gastrointest Endosc 2015;82: 425–38.

17. Tarnoff M, Rodriguez L, Escalona A, et al. Open label, prospective, randomized controlled trial of an endoscopic duodenal-jejunal bypass sleeve versus low calorie diet for pre-operative weight loss in bariatric surgery. Surg Endosc 2009;23: 650–6.

18. Schouten R, Rijs CS, Bouvy ND, et al. A multicenter, randomized efficacy study of the EndoBarrier Gastrointestinal Liner for presurgical weight loss prior to bariatric surgery. Ann Surg 2010;251:236–43.
19. de Jonge C, Rensen SS, Verdam FJ, et al. Endoscopic duodenal-jejunal bypass liner rapidly improves type 2 diabetes. Obes Surg 2013;23:1354–60.
20. GI Dynamics. GI Dynamics concludes ENDO trial. Available at: http://www.gidynamics.com/mediapress-release.php?id=148. Accessed July 30, 2015.
21. Kaplan LM, Buse JB, Mullin C, et al. EndoBarrier therapy is associated with glycemic improvement, weight loss and safety issues in patients with obesity and type 2 diabetes on oral antihyperglycemic agents. American Diabetes Association 76th Scientific Sessions. New Orleans (LA), June 12, 2016.
22. de Jonge C, Rensen SS, Koek GH, et al. Endoscopic duodenal-jejunal bypass liner rapidly improves plasma parameters of nonalcoholic fatty liver disease. Clin Gastroenterol Hepatol 2013;11:1517–20.
23. Betzel B, Koehestanie P, Aarts EO, et al. Safety experience with the duodenal-jejunal bypass liner: an endoscopic treatment for diabetes and obesity. Gastrointest Endosc 2015;82:845–52.
24. Edmundowicz S. First do no harm. Gastrointest Endosc 2015;82:853–4.
25. Betzel B, Koehestanie P, Homan J, et al. Changes in glycemic control and body weight after explantation of the duodenal-jejunal bypass liner. Gastrointest Endosc 2017;85(2):409–15.
26. Sandler B, Rumbaut R, Swain CP, et al. Human experience with an endoluminal, endoscopic, gastrojejunal bypass sleeve. Surg Endosc 2011;25:3028–33.
27. Sandler B, Rumbaut R, Swain CP, et al. One-year human experience with a novel endoluminal, endoscopic gastric bypass sleeve for morbid obesity. Surg Endosc 2015;29:3298–303.
28. Ryou M, Aihara H, Thompson CC. Minimally invasive entero-enteral dual-path bypass using self-assembling magnets. Surg Endosc 2016;30:4533–8.
29. Machytka E, Buzga M, Ryou M, et al. Endoscopic dual-path enteral anastomosis using self-assembling magnets: first-in-human clinical feasibility. Gastroenterology 2016;150(4):S232.
30. Rajagopalan H, Cherrington AD, Thompson CC, et al. Endoscopic duodenal mucosal resurfacing for the treatment of type 2 diabetes: 6-month interim analysis from the first-in-human proof-of-concept study. Diabetes Care 2016;39(12):2254–61.

Hydrothermal Duodenal Mucosal Resurfacing

Role in the Treatment of Metabolic Disease

Alan D. Cherrington, PhD[a],*, Harith Rajagopalan, MD, PhD[b],
David Maggs, MD[b], Jacques Devière, MD, PhD[c]

KEYWORDS

- Type 2 diabetes • Metabolic disease • Insulin resistance
- Nonalcoholic fatty liver disease • Duodenum • Duodenal mucosal resurfacing
- Endoscopic treatment • Hydrothermal ablation

KEY POINTS

- The dysmetabolic states of type 2 diabetes and fatty liver disease have a common pathophysiologic foundation in the form of insulin resistance, which drives end-organ disorder in beta cells and the liver respectively.
- Bariatric surgery has uncovered a potent metabolic role of the duodenum that can exert powerful effects on insulin resistance and dysmetabolic states.
- Hydrothermal duodenal mucosal resurfacing (Revita DMR) is an investigational, catheter-based, upper endoscopic procedure designed to modify signaling from the duodenal surface, thereby eliciting beneficial metabolic effects.

Continued

Disclosure Statement: A.D. Cherrington is scientific advisor/consultant to Biocon, Calibr, Eli Lilly and Company, Fractyl Laboratories, Inc, Hanmi, Islet Sciences, Merck & Co, Metavention, Novo Nordisk, NuSirt Biopharma, Profil Institute for Clinical Research, Inc, Sensulin, Thermalin Diabetes, Thetis Pharmaceuticals, vTv Therapeutics, ViaCyte, Viking, and Zafgen; receives research support from Merck & Co, Novo Nordisk, Silver Lake (1R43DK106944-01) and Galvanie; and has equity/stock options in Fractyl Laboratories, Inc, Metavention, Sensulin, LLC, Thetis Pharmaceuticals, and Zafgen. H. Rajagopalan is an employee of Fractyl Laboratories, Inc, and holds shares in the company. D. Maggs is an employee of Fractyl Laboratories, Inc, and holds shares in the company. J. Devière is a consultant for Boston Scientific, Olympus, and Cook Endoscopy and has equity in Endotools Therapeutics.

[a] Molecular Physiology & Biophysics, Vanderbilt University School of Medicine, 704A/710 Robinson Research Building, 2200 Pierce Avenue, Nashville, TN 37232-0615, USA; [b] Fractyl Laboratories, Inc, 17 Hartwell Avenue, Lexington, MA 02421, USA; [c] Medical-Surgical Department of Gastroenterology, Hepatopancreatology and Digestive Oncology, Erasme Hospital, Université Libre de Bruxelles, Route de Lennik 808, Brussels 1070, Belgium
* Corresponding author.
E-mail address: alan.cherrington@vanderbilt.edu

Continued

- Early clinical experience with hydrothermal DMR suggests that the endoscopic procedure can be safely implemented in humans, with evidence that it elicits improvements in diabetic state with potential to also affect fatty liver disease.
- Further studies are necessary to examine its clinical utility as an important treatment of the metabolic diseases that burden the modern day health care system.

INTRODUCTION

The duodenum has become increasingly recognized as a metabolic signaling center that seems to play a role in regulating insulin action and, therefore, insulin resistance states.[1–5] Insulin resistance is at the core of many dysmetabolic states, and recent advances in pharmacologic development, as well as the recognition that bariatric surgery has a major impact on glucose levels, has heightened interest in the benefits of insulin sensitization as a treatment. Data from studies of bariatric surgery and other manipulations of the upper intestine, in particular the duodenum, show that limiting nutrient exposure or contact in this key region exerts powerful metabolic effects.[1,2,6–12] Duodenal mucosal resurfacing (DMR) targets this specific biology with the assumption that the duodenal surface is in some way mediating an abnormal signal that emanates to endogenous insulin-sensitive tissues. Resurfacing through hydrothermal ablation allows a restoration of a normal mucosal interface that corrects this abnormal signal. This article describes this endoscopic approach, including the rationale for DMR and its early human use, showing its safety, tolerability, and beneficial effects on metabolism.

INSULIN-RESISTANT STATES: BACKGROUND AND CURRENT MANAGEMENT
Background

Insulin resistance is the underlying cause of several metabolic disorders, including type 2 diabetes and fatty liver disease, which affect a large segment of the general population.[13] Collectively, this pathophysiologic defect drives a massive health economic burden, manifesting with end-stage diabetes complications and premature cardiovascular disease, as well as an increasing recognition that it will also become the primary driver of end-stage liver disease.[14] Through the introduction of the insulin clamp technique in the 1970s,[15] detailed examination of the metabolic state was possible and insulin resistance was made quantifiable. This technique led to a greater understanding of the role of insulin resistance in dysmetabolic states and how insulin-sensitizing interventions exert their effects.

Lifestyle/Behavior Modification

It is recognized that lifestyle modification through healthy exercise and good nutrition can improve the metabolic state. Both lifestyle modification resulting in weight loss and the independent effects of chronic exercise reduce insulin resistance in humans. The current standard of care for treatment of type 2 diabetes promotes lifestyle and behavior modification related to exercise, weight loss, and diet before pharmacologic intervention is considered. At present, lifestyle modification is the only recognized treatment available for fatty liver disease.[16] Two landmark trials, the Diabetes Prevention Program (DPP) trial[17] and, more recently, the Look Action for Health in Diabetes (AHEAD) trial,[18,19] have shown the metabolic benefit of applying lifestyle modification in prediabetic patients and patients with frank diabetes in a controlled trial setting.

However, it is also well recognized that patients struggle to adhere to a lifestyle modification program over time and the real-world impact is transient and/or suboptimal.

Pharmacologic Treatment

Targeted treatment of insulin resistance was made available through the introduction of the thiazolidinedione (TZD) insulin-sensitizing class of agents for the treatment of type 2 diabetes.[20,21] The long-used biguanide, metformin, was also shown to have insulin-sensitizing properties at that time.[21] More recently, the glucagon-like peptide 1 receptor (GLP-1R) agonist[22] and sodium/glucose cotransporter 2 (SGLT2) inhibitor[23] classes have also been shown to have weak insulin-sensitizing properties, which may or may not have a weight-independent component.

It was through the use of these pharmacologic agents in the clinic that a wider array of their effects was observed beyond improved glycemic control: reductions in blood pressure, lowering of hepatic transaminase levels, altered lipid metabolism, and restoration of ovulation in previously anovulatory women with features of the insulin-resistant condition polycystic ovarian syndrome (PCOS; also termed metabolic reproductive syndrome). These effects allowed a broader view of insulin action and insulin-sensitive end-organs (ie, liver, skeletal muscle, adipose tissue, ovary) and how they are each affected by insulin resistance. Metformin, the TZDs and GLP-1r agonists have each shown positive attributes in one or more insulin-sensitive end-organ systems beyond their ability to improve glycemia. More specifically, both TZDs and GLP-1r agonists have been explored in fatty liver disease,[24] and metformin, TZDs, and GLP-1r agonists have shown positive effects in patients with PCOS.[25]

However, although pharmacologic intervention has brought a broad array of benefits through insulin sensitization, a major drawback of these agents has been the ability of patients to adhere to regular daily dosing,[26] which is related in part to these agents' unattractive side effects, including gastrointestinal intolerance (metformin and GLP1r agonists), edema (TZDs) and heart failure (TZDs). In the case of GLP-1r agonists, route of administration (ie, injection) may also pose a barrier.

Bariatric Surgery

Over the last 20 years, bariatric surgery involving bypass of the upper intestine has become established as a highly impactful intervention that elicits beneficial metabolic effects. It has been shown to result in dramatic improvements in the glycemic state and so-called disease remission in some patients with type 2 diabetes.[27] It has also been shown to halt or reverse disease progression of nonalcoholic steatohepatitis (NASH),[10] and to correct anovulation in PCOS.[28] The groundswell of interest in surgery and its metabolic effects has resulted in the recent authoring of a consensus statement, embraced by multiple professional organizations, recommending that bariatric (now termed metabolic) surgeries be included in the treatment algorithm for patients with type 2 diabetes.[9] It is notable that much of the metabolic benefit is observed acutely, within days of the procedure, preceding by weeks and months the substantial weight loss that is also seen with bariatric surgery.[29–31] This effect is noted particularly after Roux en Y gastric bypass, suggesting that avoiding the contact of food with the duodenum and proximal jejunum may quickly elicit beneficial metabolic effects. More recently, detailed accounts of metabolic changes by various investigators have shown that there is a clear and measurable insulin-sensitizing effect within the first 2 weeks postsurgery that is sustained over time (a year or more).[29,31–33] The insulin-sensitizing response seems to be an important contributor to the observed metabolic effect, and it is hard to consider either short-term caloric restriction as a consequence of the surgery or a surgery-mediated incretin effect to be a major confounder of this observation. As further evidence of the substantial regulatory role this gut-borne signal apparently plays in diabetic rats and humans with type 2 diabetes, reintroduction of nutrients to the bypassed section of duodenum rapidly elicits a return to hyperglycemia and restores insulin resistance.[34,35]

The duodenal-jejunal bypass sleeve (or EndoBarrier GI liner [GI Dynamics, Inc, Boston, MA]) gives further credence to the mechanism observed with bariatric surgery. The sleeve is anchored in the duodenal bulb and prevents contact of food with the mucosal surface of the duodenum and proximal jejunum. The implanted sleeve device is placed for up to 12 months in situ and it has been shown to induce some weight loss in obese patients and to improve glucose homeostasis in patients with type 2 diabetes.[36–38]

Bariatric surgery is likely to remain a key component of the type 2 diabetes treatment algorithm and, as more data accumulate, it may establish a therapeutic role in fatty liver disease and other dysmetabolic states, and even more so as technological and surgical techniques advance. However, bariatric surgery is unlikely to become a major solution at a population level, because it is not an easily scalable intervention and surgery remains a disincentive for many patients.

METABOLIC ROLE OF THE DUODENUM

An increasing body of evidence suggests that the duodenum is a key metabolic signaling center and the mucosal surface may manifest with some form of maladaptation when exposed to unhealthy nutrients through fat and sugar ingestion. These changes imply a role of the duodenum in the development of insulin resistance and the pathogenesis of related metabolic diseases.

Evidence from Animal Models

In animal studies, researchers have described both morphologic and functional changes in the duodenum following unhealthy nutrient exposure. Adachi and colleagues[39] reported morphologic changes in the small intestines of 3 types of diabetic rats and observed intestinal hyperplasia in all of the models. These researchers also showed that markers of proliferation were increased in diabetic strains compared with controls. In the Wistar rat, Gniuli and colleagues[40] found that a high-fat diet stimulates duodenal proliferation of endocrine cells differentiating toward K cells and oversecreting gastric inhibitory polypeptide (GIP). Bailey and colleagues[41] showed in obese hyperglycemic (ob/ob) mice that a high-fat diet stimulates the production and secretion of intestinal immunoreactive GIP, a mediator of insulin secretion, and increases the density of GIP-secreting intestinal K cells compared with a stock diet. Ponter and colleagues[42] have similarly shown alterations in plasma and small intestinal GIP in response to a high-fat diet in pigs.

Lee and colleagues[43] observed impaired glucose sensing in the enteroendocrine and enterochromaffin cells in a diabetic rodent model, with evidence of impaired downstream neural signaling in the gut.

Salinari and colleagues[44] tested the effects of proteins extracted from the duodenum-jejunum conditioned-medium of db/db (diabetic) or Swiss (nondiabetic) mice, or from the jejunum of insulin-resistant human subjects captured during abdominal surgery. The mouse proteins were tested in several experimental settings, including in vivo in Swiss mice during an intraperitoneal caloric challenge, and in Swiss mice soleus muscle in vitro, whereas human-extracted proteins were studied on human myotubes ex vivo. Overall, these proteins were found to cause insulin resistance in cultured muscle cells, whether of murine or human origin, providing strong evidence that a factor isolated from the duodenal or jejunal tissue may affect insulin sensitivity.

Evidence from Humans

In concert with animal findings, studies in humans also reveal abnormal mucosal hypertrophy, hyperplasia of enteroendocrine cells, and increases in enteroendocrine cell and enterocyte numbers in the upper GI tracts of diabetic patients compared with nondiabetic controls.[3,5]

Theodorakis and colleagues[3] specifically noted an increase in L and L/K cells in the duodenal mucosa of type 2 diabetic patients compared with nondiabetic controls, whereas Verdam and colleagues[5] showed increases in small intestinal enterocyte mass and increases in enterocyte loss related to chronic hyperglycemia in severely obese subjects. Salinari and colleagues[12] conducted an intricate study of the upper GI tract in obese subjects with and without type 2 diabetes by infusing nutrients at 3 different starting points in the small bowel (duodenum, proximal jejunum, and mid-jejunum) through a balloon catheter. They showed that bypass of the duodenum, with delivery of nutrients to the jejunum instead, resulted in an approximate 50% increase in insulin sensitivity in both groups. This finding offers direct evidence of the apparent insulin-resisting signal that seems to emanate from the region of the duodenum and how it is attenuated when nutrient delivery to the region is prevented.

DUODENAL MUCOSAL RESURFACING: METHOD FOR CORRECTING DUODENAL METABOLIC SIGNALING
Rationale for Targeting Duodenal Mucosa

Collectively, the observations described earlier support an approach that targets the duodenum mucosal surface for the treatment of metabolic disease without the need for placing a permanent implant. To this end, a novel endoscopic catheter system (Revita DMR system [Fractyl Laboratories, Inc, Lexington, MA]) was designed to deliver a hydrothermal exchange at the mucosal surface, resulting in superficial tissue ablation. Currently under investigation in the United States, the Revita DMR system holds a CE (Conformité Européene) mark in Europe.

As background, ablation is a common treatment modality for a wide variety of medical conditions (**Table 1**). Intervention involves the physical removal of superficial abnormal tissue and the regrowth and restoration of normal tissue through a stem cell–mediated healing response. The most anatomically analogous approach to DMR is endoscopic ablative therapy through either radiofrequency (Barrx, Covidien, Sunnyvale, CA) or argon plasma coagulation for Barrett's esophagus, a precancerous condition and complication of gastroesophageal reflux disease, in which the normal squamous epithelium of the distal esophagus transforms to a columnar-lined intestinal metaplasia.[45,46] This treatment modality has become well established and its efficacy and safety are well described.[47] Ablation is followed by restoration of the squamous epithelium.[48]

Targeting Duodenal Mucosa in Animal Models: Proof of Concept

As described by Rajagopalan and colleagues,[60] Revita DMR was first explored in preclinical rodent and porcine models. In diabetic rats (Goto-Kakizaki), selective denudation of the duodenal mucosa conducted by an abrasion device improved

Table 1
Examples of ablation methods and their clinical applications

Ablation Method	Examples of Clinical Use
Radiofrequency	Barrett's esophagus[46]
	Atrial fibrillation[49]
	Liver tumors[50]
Laser	Benign prostatic hyperplasia[51]
	Dermatologic conditions[52]
Cryoablation	Atrial fibrillation[49]
	Actinic keratosis[53]
	Warts[54]
Chemical	Cardiac arrhythmias[55]
	Telangiectasias[56]
	Facial rejuvenation[57]
Mechanical	Dermatologic conditions[58]
Hydrothermal	Heavy uterine bleeding[59]
	Type 2 diabetes (investigational [United States], approved [European Union])[60]
	NAFLD/NASH (investigational)[61]

Abbreviation: NAFLD, nonalcoholic fatty liver disease.

glucose tolerance compared with preprocedure tolerance and also compared with sham-treated diabetic controls (**Fig. 1**). Of note, in nondiabetic (Sprague-Dawley) rodents that received the same treatment, there was no improvement in glucose tolerance. These findings suggest that this duodenum-directed intervention was effective in treating abnormal hyperglycemia, but without an effect in normal animals. Subsequent safety studies conducted in a porcine model showed that hydrothermal ablation was feasible and, when applied as described, was limited to the superficial intestinal mucosa and did not damage the underlying muscularis mucosa or deeper structures (Rajagopalan H et al, unpublished data, Fractyl Laboratories, Inc, Lexington, MA).

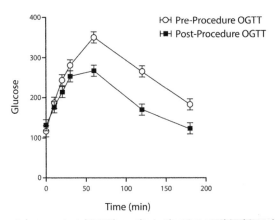

Fig. 1. Oral glucose tolerance test (OGTT) results in the Goto-Kakizaki rat (n = 9) before and after duodenal abrasion. Duodenal abrasion was associated with a 25% improvement in area under the curve for OGTT.

Duodenal Mucosal Resurfacing Catheter (Revita) and Procedure

DMR is an upper endoscopic, catheter-based procedure that uses a combination of circumferential mucosal lift (via a homogeneous submucosal injection, separating superficial mucosa from underlying muscularis) of the target segment of duodenum and hydrothermal ablation via a novel, wire-guided balloon catheter system (**Fig. 2**). This ablation is followed by a re-epithelialization of the treated duodenal lumen that seems to initiate fairly immediately, within days following procedure, achieving a reset of duodenal mucosa in patients with type 2 diabetes.

The procedure is performed on patients under general anesthesia with a duration of just less than 60 minutes. The catheter is used to first size the duodenum and then circumferentially lift the mucosa from the underlying muscularis with saline submucosal injection to provide a uniform ablative surface and a thermally protective layer of saline between the mucosa and deeper tissue layers. Under direct endoscopic visualization, discrete circumferential hydrothermal ablations lasting approximately 10 seconds each are applied at temperatures of approximately 90°C, with the goal of obtaining up to 5 longitudinally separated ablations along a length of approximately 9 to 10 cm of post-papillary duodenum (**Fig. 3**). The procedure is performed starting at the post-papilla and ending proximal to the ligament of Treitz. It is monitored and controlled by the physician from a stand-alone console. In the 24 hours postprocedure, patients are able to resume an oral diet but are counseled to adhere to a puree/semisolid diet for the next 10 to 14 days without an intended caloric restriction.

First-in-Human Study of Revita Duodenal Mucosal Resurfacing in Type 2 Diabetes

Six-month safety and efficacy data from a single-arm, open-label, nonrandomized, first-in-human (FIH) study of Revita DMR has recently been published.[60] At the time of the report the study, performed at a single site in South America, had enrolled 44 patients with type 2 diabetes who were poorly controlled and were on at least 1 oral antidiabetic medication. At screening, patients had hemoglobin A1c (HbA1c) levels that ranged from 7.5% to 12% (average of 9.5%). Enrolled patients ranged in age from 38 to 65 years, had type 2 diabetes for a duration of less than 10 years, and were overweight or obese as defined by body mass index (average, 30.8 kg/m^2). Patients on injectable medications, including insulin, were excluded from participation.

Safety Profile of Duodenal Mucosal Resurfacing in Early Human Use

Of the original patient cohort, the DMR procedure was completed without periprocedural complication in all 40 treated patients and was well tolerated. There was no

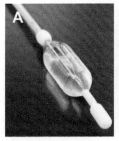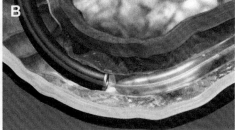

Fig. 2. Revita DMR catheter. (*A*) First-generation, single-use balloon catheter used to perform hydrothermal ablation of the duodenal mucosa. (*B*) The balloon inflated in the duodenum during hydrothermal ablation. (*Courtesy of* Fractyl Laboratories, Inc, Lexington, MA; with permission.)

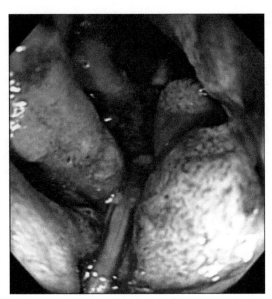

Fig. 3. The duodenal mucosa immediately after hydrothermal ablation. (*Courtesy of* Fractyl Laboratories, Inc, Lexington, MA; with permission.)

observed bleeding, perforation, infection, or pancreatitis. In addition, there were no obvious features of malabsorption (as indicated by hematological and chemistry measures) and DMR did not seem to cause hypoglycemia. The most common study-related adverse event was mild, transient, postprocedural abdominal pain in 20% of patients (8 out of 40) that resolved without treatment within 48 hours. Follow-up endoscopies and duodenal biopsies in a subset of patients from the FIH study showed mucosal healing in all evaluated patients. Three patients had procedure-related duodenal stenosis, which was successfully treated by single nonemergent endoscopic balloon dilation in each case without further complications. In total, 90 DMR procedures have been conducted thus far with no further stenosis cases since those reported in the original cohort.

Glycemic Improvement in Subjects with Type 2 Diabetes in the First-in-Human Study

In the FIH 6-month interim report, DMR elicited a decrease of glycemia that was prompt (in the first 1–2 weeks) and resulted in significant lowering of HbA1c levels (**Fig. 4**A). It was also observed that subjects who had longer segment ablation (average length, ~9 cm) showed a greater glycemic improvement than those subjects who had a shorter segment ablation (~3 cm), thus indicating an ablation dose dependency. Closer assessment showed that most of the plasma glucose level lowering was a reflection of fasting glucose reduction (~40–50 mg/dL), suggesting a predominant impact on overnight basal hepatic production. There was nonetheless a small additional reduction of the postprandial glycemic excursion contributing to the overall effect. There was some rebound or loss of glycemic effect observed in certain patients at 6 months, but this observation was confounded by a reduction in background medication in many. For patients who remained on stable medication postprocedure, there seemed to be a greater reduction in HbA1c level at 6 months (−1.8%) and better durability of the glycemic effect than in patients whose medications were changed during the course of the study. This improvement in glycemic state was accompanied by a

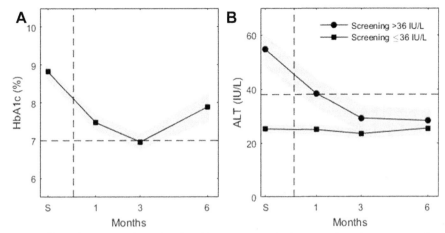

Fig. 4. Effect of DMR on HbA1c level and liver enzymes in the FIH cohort (most recent data capture of n = 48). Shaded area is ±1 standard error of the mean. (*A*) HbA1c levels at screening, 1, 3, and 6 months in subjects with preprocedure HbA1c levels of 7.5% to 10% and 3 or more ablations (n = 19). (*B*) Impact of DMR on alanine transaminase (ALT) by screening ALT level in subjects with 3 or more ablations (highest screening ALT, n = 15; lowest screening ALT, n = 15).

significant lowering of HOMA-IR (Homeostatic Model Assessment of Insulin Resistance) as an indicator of improved insulin sensitivity (Rajagopalan H et al, unpublished data, Fractyl Laboratories, Inc, Lexington, MA). Of note, there was a modest effect on body weight during the 6 months, with a ~3-kg weight loss noted at 3 months and a return toward preprocedure weight by 6 months, suggesting that the effect was unlikely to be explained by alterations in body weight.

Wider Metabolic Effects of Duodenal Mucosal Resurfacing Observed in Human Subjects

As described with insulin-sensitizing pharmacologic approaches (eg, TZD) and bariatric surgery, a wider array of metabolic effects could be anticipated with DMR. In the FIH study, a lowering of hepatic transaminase levels from preprocedure values was observed, and the reductions were more striking in subjects with higher preprocedure levels (**Fig. 4B**). In the patients receiving long-segment ablation (n = 28), both alanine transaminase (ALT) and aspartate transaminase (AST) levels were reduced by approximately 30% at 6 months.[61] Moreover, reductions in ALT and AST were also seen in a subset of patients from the FIH study who had incidental findings of fatty liver on ultrasonography examination in the months before procedure. Although these findings are preliminary, further study of liver indices (including circulating, radiological, elastographic, and tissue indices) in patients post-DMR are warranted to determine whether DMR has an important impact on fatty liver disease pathophysiology. In addition, in anticipation of other apparent insulin-sensitizing effects, assessment of DMR effects on cardiovascular (ie, blood pressure, microalbumin) indices and ovulatory function in women are necessary.

SUMMARY

Early human clinical trial data suggest that endoscopic hydrothermal DMR ablation is well tolerated in humans with an acceptable safety profile thus far. This novel, single-point procedure elicits an improvement in the metabolic state through substantial reductions in glycemia in patients with poorly controlled type 2 diabetes. Preliminary data also suggest an improvement of hepatic transaminase levels when increased before treatment. These findings underscore the notion of the duodenum as an important metabolic signaling center that plays a role in regulating insulin sensitivity. As westernized countries face an increasing economic health burden from diseases driven by insulin resistance (eg, diabetes, fatty liver disease, cardiovascular disease) and the shortcomings of lifestyle, pharmacologic, and surgical approaches limit their applicability and efficacy, this novel endoscopic treatment approach may offer an important alternative for patients. Further studies are necessary to understand the core mechanism, how the procedure performs in a randomized clinical trial setting, and the duration of the beneficial effect, while also embracing the potential for wider metabolic benefits.

REFERENCES

1. Rubino F, Forgione A, Cummings DE, et al. The mechanism of diabetes control after gastrointestinal bypass surgery reveals a role of the proximal small intestine in the pathophysiology of type 2 diabetes. Ann Surg 2006;244(5):741–9.
2. Zervos EE, Agle SC, Warren AJ, et al. Amelioration of insulin requirement in patients undergoing duodenal bypass for reasons other than obesity implicates foregut factors in the pathophysiology of type II diabetes. J Am Coll Surg 2010 May;210(5):564–72, 572–4.
3. Theodorakis MJ, Carlson O, Michopoulos S, et al. Human duodenal enteroendocrine cells: source of both incretin peptides, GLP-1 and GIP. Am J Physiol Endocrinol Metab 2006;290(3):E550–9.
4. Nguyen NQ, Debreceni TL, Bambrick JE, et al. Accelerated intestinal glucose absorption in morbidly obese humans: relationship to glucose transporters, incretin hormones, and glycemia. J Clin Endocrinol Metab 2015;100(3):968–76.
5. Verdam FJ, Greve JWM, Roosta S, et al. Small intestinal alterations in severely obese hyperglycemic subjects. J Clin Endocrinol Metab 2011;96(2):E379–83.
6. de Jonge C, Rensen SS, Verdam FJ, et al. Endoscopic duodenal-jejunal bypass liner rapidly improves type 2 diabetes. Obes Surg 2013;23(9):1354–60.
7. Laferrère B, Reilly D, Arias S, et al. Differential metabolic impact of gastric bypass surgery versus dietary intervention in obese diabetic subjects despite identical weight loss. Sci Transl Med 2011;3(80):80re2.
8. Rubino F, R'bibo SL, del Genio F, et al. Metabolic surgery: the role of the gastrointestinal tract in diabetes mellitus. Nat Rev Endocrinol 2010;6(2):102–9.
9. Rubino F, Nathan DM, Eckel RH, et al. Metabolic surgery in the treatment algorithm for type 2 diabetes: a joint statement by international diabetes organizations. Diabetes Care 2016;39(6):861–77.
10. Caiazzo R, Lassailly G, Leteurtre E, et al. Roux-en-Y gastric bypass versus adjustable gastric banding to reduce nonalcoholic fatty liver disease: a 5-year controlled longitudinal study. Ann Surg 2014;260(5):893–8 [discussion: 898–9].
11. Zhang X, Xiao Z, Yu H, et al. Short-term glucose metabolism and gut hormone modulations after Billroth II gastrojejunostomy in nonobese gastric cancer patients with type 2 diabetes mellitus, impaired glucose tolerance and normal glucose tolerance. Arch Med Res 2013;44(6):437–43.
12. Salinari S, Carr RD, Guidone C, et al. Nutrient infusion bypassing duodenum-jejunum improves insulin sensitivity in glucose-tolerant and diabetic obese subjects. Am J Physiol Endocrinol Metab 2013;305(1):E59–66.

13. Saponaro C, Gaggini M, Gastaldelli A. Nonalcoholic fatty liver disease and type 2 diabetes: common pathophysiologic mechanisms. Curr Diab Rep 2015;15(6):607.
14. Calzadilla Bertot L, Adams LA. The natural course of non-alcoholic fatty liver disease. Int J Mol Sci 2016;17(5) [pii:E774].
15. DeFronzo RA, Tobin JD, Andres R. Glucose clamp technique: a method for quantifying insulin secretion and resistance. Am J Physiol 1979;237(3):E214–23.
16. Rotman Y, Sanyal AJ. Current and upcoming pharmacotherapy for non-alcoholic fatty liver disease. Gut 2016. http://dx.doi.org/10.1136/gutjnl-2016-312431.
17. Knowler WC, Barrett-Connor E, Fowler SE, et al. Reduction in the incidence of type 2 diabetes with lifestyle intervention or metformin. N Engl J Med 2002; 346(6):393–403.
18. Dutton GR, Lewis CE. The Look AHEAD trial: Implications for lifestyle intervention in type 2 diabetes mellitus. Prog Cardiovasc Dis 2015;58(1):69–75.
19. Look AHEAD Research Group, Wing RR, Bolin P, et al. Cardiovascular effects of intensive lifestyle intervention in type 2 diabetes. N Engl J Med 2013;369(2): 145–54.
20. Lefèbvre PJ, Scheen AJ. Improving the action of insulin. Clin Investig Med 1995; 18(4):340–7.
21. Inzucchi SE, Maggs DG, Spollett GR, et al. Efficacy and metabolic effects of metformin and troglitazone in type II diabetes mellitus. N Engl J Med 1998;338(13): 867–72.
22. DeFronzo RA, Triplitt C, Qu Y, et al. Effects of exenatide plus rosiglitazone on beta-cell function and insulin sensitivity in subjects with type 2 diabetes on metformin. Diabetes Care 2010;33(5):951–7.
23. Daniele G, Xiong J, Solis-Herrera C, et al. Dapagliflozin enhances fat oxidation and ketone production in patients with type 2 diabetes. Diabetes Care 2016. http://dx.doi.org/10.2337/dc15-2688.
24. Barb D, Portillo-Sanchez P, Cusi K, et al. Pharmacological management of nonalcoholic fatty liver disease. Metabolism 2016;65(8):1183–95.
25. Elkind-Hirsch K, Marrioneaux O, Bhushan M, et al. Comparison of single and combined treatment with exenatide and metformin on menstrual cyclicity in overweight women with polycystic ovary syndrome. J Clin Endocrinol Metab 2008; 93(7):2670–8.
26. Inzucchi SE, Bergenstal RM, Buse JB, et al. Management of hyperglycemia in type 2 diabetes, 2015: a patient-centered approach: update to a position statement of the American Diabetes Association and the European Association for the Study of Diabetes. Diabetes Care 2014;38(1):140–9.
27. Ferrannini E, Mingrone G. Impact of different bariatric surgical procedures on insulin action and beta-cell function in type 2 diabetes. Diabetes Care 2009;32(3): 514–20.
28. Skubleny D, Switzer NJ, Gill RS, et al. The impact of bariatric surgery on polycystic ovary syndrome: a systematic review and meta-analysis. Obes Surg 2016; 26(1):169–76.
29. Umeda LM, Silva EA, Carneiro G, et al. Early improvement in glycemic control after bariatric surgery and its relationships with insulin, GLP-1, and glucagon secretion in type 2 diabetic patients. Obes Surg 2011;21(7):896–901.
30. Jacobsen SH, Olesen SC, Dirksen C, et al. Changes in gastrointestinal hormone responses, insulin sensitivity, and beta-cell function within 2 weeks after gastric bypass in non-diabetic subjects. Obes Surg 2012;22(7):1084–96.
31. Bojsen-Møller KN, Dirksen C, Jørgensen NB, et al. Early enhancements of hepatic and later of peripheral insulin sensitivity combined with increased postprandial

insulin secretion contribute to improved glycemic control after Roux-en-Y gastric bypass. Diabetes 2014;63(5):1725–37.

32. Bikman BT, Zheng D, Pories WJ, et al. Mechanism for improved insulin sensitivity after gastric bypass surgery. J Clin Endocrinol Metab 2008;93(12):4656–63.

33. Jørgensen NB, Jacobsen SH, Dirksen C, et al. Acute and long-term effects of Roux-en-Y gastric bypass on glucose metabolism in subjects with type 2 diabetes and normal glucose tolerance. Am J Physiol Endocrinol Metab 2012; 303(1):E122–31.

34. Dirksen C, Hansen DL, Madsbad S, et al. Postprandial diabetic glucose tolerance is normalized by gastric bypass feeding as opposed to gastric feeding and is associated with exaggerated GLP-1 secretion: a case report. Diabetes Care 2010;33(2):375–7.

35. Shimizu H, Eldar S, Heneghan HM, et al. The effect of selective gut stimulation on glucose metabolism after gastric bypass in the Zucker diabetic fatty rat model. Surg Obes Relat Dis 2014;10(1):29–35.

36. Rohde U, Hedbäck N, Gluud LL, et al. Effect of the EndoBarrier gastrointestinal liner on obesity and type 2 diabetes: a systematic review and meta-analysis. Diabetes Obes Metab 2016;18(3):300–5.

37. Rohde U, Federspiel CA, Vilmann P, et al. The impact of EndoBarrier gastrointestinal liner in obese patients with normal glucose tolerance and patients with type 2 diabetes. Diabetes Obes Metab 2016. http://dx.doi.org/10.1111/dom.12800.

38. Vilarrasa N, de Gordejuela AGR, Casajoana A, et al. EndoBarrier in grade I obese patients with long-standing type 2 diabetes: role of gastrointestinal hormones in glucose metabolism. Obes Surg 2016. http://dx.doi.org/10.1007/s11695-016-2311-0.

39. Adachi T, Mori C, Sakurai K, et al. Morphological changes and increased sucrase and isomaltase activity in small intestines of insulin-deficient and type 2 diabetic rats. Endocr J 2003;50(3):271–9.

40. Gniuli D, Calcagno A, Dalla Libera L, et al. High-fat feeding stimulates endocrine, glucose-dependent insulinotropic polypeptide (GIP)-expressing cell hyperplasia in the duodenum of Wistar rats. Diabetologia 2010;53(10):2233–40.

41. Bailey CJ, Flatt PR, Kwasowski P, et al. Immunoreactive gastric inhibitory polypeptide and K cell hyperplasia in obese hyperglycaemic (ob/ob) mice fed high fat and high carbohydrate cafeteria diets. Acta Endocrinol (Copenh) 1986; 112(2):224–9.

42. Ponter AA, Salter DN, Morgan LM, et al. The effect of energy source and feeding level on the hormones of the entero-insular axis and plasma glucose in the growing pig. Br J Nutr 1991;66(2):187–97.

43. Lee J, Cummings BP, Martin E, et al. Glucose sensing by gut endocrine cells and activation of the vagal afferent pathway is impaired in a rodent model of type 2 diabetes mellitus. Am J Physiol Regul Integr Comp Physiol 2012;302(6):R657–66.

44. Salinari S, Debard C, Bertuzzi A, et al. Jejunal proteins secreted by db/db mice or insulin-resistant humans impair the insulin signaling and determine insulin resistance. PLoS One 2013;8(2):e56258.

45. Kalatskaya I. Overview of major molecular alterations during progression from Barrett's esophagus to esophageal adenocarcinoma. Ann N Y Acad Sci 2016. http://dx.doi.org/10.1111/nyas.13134.

46. Peter S, Mönkemüller K. Ablative endoscopic therapies for Barrett's-esophagus-related neoplasia. Gastroenterol Clin North Am 2015;44(2):337–53.

47. Qumseya BJ, Wani S, Desai M, et al. Adverse events after radiofrequency ablation in patients with Barrett's esophagus: a systematic review and meta-analysis. Clin Gastroenterol Hepatol 2016;14(8):1086–95.e6.
48. Berenson MM, Johnson TD, Markowitz NR, et al. Restoration of squamous mucosa after ablation of Barrett's esophageal epithelium. Gastroenterology 1993; 104(6):1686–91.
49. Jiang J, Li J, Zhong G, et al. Efficacy and safety of the second-generation cryoballoons versus radiofrequency ablation for the treatment of paroxysmal atrial fibrillation: a systematic review and meta-analysis. J Interv Card Electrophysiol 2016. http://dx.doi.org/10.1007/s10840-016-0191-9.
50. Meyer J, Toomay S. Update on treatment of liver metastases: focus on ablation therapies. Curr Oncol Rep 2015;17(1):420.
51. Nair SM, Pimentel MA, Gilling PJ. A review of laser treatment for symptomatic BPH (benign prostatic hyperplasia). Curr Urol Rep 2016;17(6):45.
52. Yates B, Que SKT, D'Souza L, et al. Laser treatment of periocular skin conditions. Clin Dermatol 2015;33(2):197–206.
53. Peris K, Fargnoli MC. Conventional treatment of actinic keratosis: an overview. Curr Probl Dermatol 2015;46:108–14.
54. Zimmerman EE, Crawford P. Cutaneous cryosurgery. Am Fam Physician 2012; 86(12):1118–24.
55. Schurmann P, Peñalver J, Valderrábano M. Ethanol for the treatment of cardiac arrhythmias. Curr Opin Cardiol 2015;30(4):333–43.
56. Schwartz L, Maxwell H. Sclerotherapy for lower limb telangiectasias. Cochrane Database Syst Rev 2011;(12):CD008826.
57. Meaike JD, Agrawal N, Chang D, et al. Noninvasive facial rejuvenation. Part 3: Physician-directed-lasers, chemical peels, and other noninvasive modalities. Semin Plast Surg 2016;30(3):143–50.
58. Gozali MV, Zhou B. Effective treatments of atrophic acne scars. J Clin Aesthet Dermatol 2015;8(5):33–40.
59. Fernandez H. Update on the management of menometrorrhagia: new surgical approaches. Gynecol Endocrinol 2011;27(Suppl 1):1131–6.
60. Rajagopalan H, Cherrington AD, Thompson CC, et al. Endoscopic duodenal mucosal resurfacing for the treatment of type 2 diabetes: 6-month interim analysis from the first-in-human proof-of-concept study. Diabetes Care 2016. http://dx.doi.org/10.2337/dc16-0383.
61. Neto MG, Rajagopalan H, Becerra P, et al. 829 Endoscopic duodenal mucosal resurfacing improves glycemic and hepatic parameters in patients with type 2 diabetes: data from a first-in-human study. Gastroenterology 2016;150(4):S174.

Therapeutic Options to Treat Pediatric Obesity

Allen F. Browne, MD, Diplomate ABOM*

KEYWORDS

- Obesity • Pediatric • Children • Adolescent • Pharmacotherapy
- Medical device therapy • Endoscopic therapy • Bariatric surgery

KEY POINTS

- Obesity in children and adolescents is a severe health, psychosocial, and economic problem.
- Treatment of obesity should be based on the physiology, biochemistry, and genetics of the disease.
- The foundation of treatment of obesity should be a healthy environment, including healthy eating, healthy activity, and mental health support.
- Patients with obesity usually need more than diet, activity, and behavior to control their disease.
- The most successful treatment of obesity follows a chronic disease model, provides a continuum of care, and involves many different disciplines.

INTRODUCTION

The need for effective treatment of obese children and adolescents is increasingly agreed on. Clinicians now recognize that a significant percentage of children and adolescents with obesity become obese adults. They also have significant psychosocial and medical comorbidities while they are children as well as when they become adults. As the physiology and biochemistry of obesity is being unraveled, it becomes apparent that obesity is not a voluntary behavior problem on the part of the pediatric patient or their parents. Obesity is the energy regulatory system of the body gone awry and driving unhealthy behavior. Obesity is the root cause of many comorbidities. These comorbidities prevent a healthy life, a high-quality life, and a productive life. Comorbidities result in massive health care costs throughout the lifetime of the patient.[1,2] There is now strong evidence of the effectiveness of a multidisciplinary

Disclosure Statement: The author has nothing to disclose.
Department of Surgery, Maine Medical Center, 22 Bramhall Street, Portland, ME 04102, USA
* 25 Andrews Avenue, Falmouth, ME 04105.
E-mail address: allenbrowne@sbcglobal.net

Gastrointest Endoscopy Clin N Am 27 (2017) 313–326
http://dx.doi.org/10.1016/j.giec.2017.01.003
1052-5157/17/© 2017 Elsevier Inc. All rights reserved.

giendo.theclinics.com

approach to obesity leading to an improved quality of life, resolution of comorbidities, improved economic productivity, and decreased health care costs.[3–7]

This article:

1. Discusses the goals of therapy when treating pediatric obesity
2. Presents the basic cornerstones of diet, activity, and behavior that need to be provided to all pediatric patients with obesity and their families
3. Presents bariatric procedures that have been shown to help adolescent and pediatric patients with obesity
4. Speculates how weight loss medications might be used to help pediatric patients with obesity
5. Speculates how weight loss devices might be used to help pediatric patients with obesity
6. Speculates how endoscopic weight loss procedures might be used to help pediatric patients with obesity
7. Speculates how some theoretic techniques might be used to help pediatric patients with obesity

Gastroenterologists might be involved in pediatric weight management in many ways:

1. As obesity medicine specialists directing the multidisciplinary weight management program
2. In the care of obesity-related comorbidities such as nonalcoholic fatty liver disease
3. Using endoscopic skills to revise bariatric procedures
4. Performing endoscopic versions of bariatric procedures
5. Placing, adjusting, and removing weight loss devices

GOALS OF THERAPY

The goals of therapy for pediatric patients with obesity include improving the quality of life, resolution and/or prevention of comorbidities, improving economic productivity when patients become adults, and reducing lifetime health care costs.

Identification and objective measurement of childhood obesity are accomplished by calculating body mass index (BMI) for age and gender. Although percentage body fat is a better measure of obesity and the accompanying visual, metabolic, and physiologic issues, it is more difficult and expensive to do, and thus is not commonly done.

BMI charts for age and gender are readily available.[8] Using the child's height, weight, age, and gender, the patient can be categorized on the appropriate growth chart (**Table 1**).

With a child increasing in height and age, keeping a stable weight may result in an improvement in the classification of the obesity. Calculating the predicted ultimate adult height for a child with obesity provides information on whether weight loss will

Table 1	
Pediatric body mass index categories	
BMI Category	**BMI Percentile**
Overweight	>85th percentile to <95th percentile
Obesity: class 1	>95th percentile to <120% of the 95th percentile
Obesity: class 2	120% to <140% of the 95th percentile or BMI 35 to <40 (whichever is lower)
Obesity: class 3	>140% of the 95th percentile or BMI >40 (whichever is lower)

be necessary or how much weight loss might be necessary to reach a normal BMI. The raw BMI or the BMI percentile for age and gender when the BMI is more than the 95th percentile is no longer appropriate.[9] The categorization system mentioned earlier allows better monitoring. How aggressively to attempt to return a given patient to a normal BMI percentile is still an open question, but BMI percentile for age and gender is very useful to follow each patient's progress.

Although BMI is convenient and useful, evaluation of psychosocial and clinical comorbidities is ultimately more important. There are pediatric weight-related quality-of-life scales that can be used to identify and follow psychosocial comorbidities and the progress of the patient.[10] Monitoring children for bullying and stigmatization episodes, depression, and other mental health issues is standard of care (**Box 1**).[11]

Evaluation for clinical comorbidities involves testing for subclinical and clinical disease as well as risk factors for clinical comorbidities (**Table 2**).

When abnormalities are found, they need to be monitored. In addition, a general evaluation should be performed at regular intervals to screen for additional clinical and psychosocial comorbidities. Reaching the goal of improving or eliminating psychosocial and clinical comorbidities is more important than reaching a normal BMI.

DIET, ACTIVITY, AND BEHAVIOR: HEALTHY LIVING

Healthy living is the cornerstone on which all other weight management therapies and tools are based. A pediatric weight management program providing various advanced therapeutic options must have personnel who are trained and skilled in the management of diet, activity, and behavior.

The blueprint for the application of diet, activity, and behavior is outlined in the 2007 AAP recommendations, "Expert Committee Recommendations Regarding the Prevention, Assessment and Treatment of Child and Adolescent Overweight and Obesity: Summary Report."[12] These recommendations show an increasing frequency and intensity of assessment and education from stages 1 through 4. Stages 1 and 2 are delivered in primary care offices. Stage 3 involves specialists in the treatment of children with obesity and brings up the possibility of pharmacotherapy. Stage 4 continues the work by specialists in obesity medicine and brings up the possibility of bariatric surgery. In the advanced stages (3 and 4), a multidisciplinary team that includes a dietitian, an activity specialist, and a behavior health specialist is advised.[12] The progression from one stage to the next is based on response to therapy. The weight goals vary with the age of the patient and the stage of disease.[12]

In general, the success of healthy living practices is marginal.[13–16] However, measurements of success are hampered by lack of agreement on goals. Some studies

---

Box 1
Evaluation for psychosocial comorbidities

Depression

Quality of life

School performance

Adverse childhood experiences

Bullying experiences

Table 2
Evaluation for clinical comorbidities

Clinical Disease	Subclinical Disease	Risk Factors for Future Comorbidities
Type 2 diabetes	Insulin resistance	Metabolic syndrome
Asthma	Nonalcoholic fatty liver disease	Dyslipidemia
Hypertension		Left ventricular hypertrophy
Sleep apnea		
Gastroesophageal reflux disease		
Orthopedic disorders		
Polycystic ovary syndrome		
Pseudotumor cerebri		

emphasize BMI, others emphasize comorbidities, whereas others try to extrapolate to future risk of disease. There is general agreement that advanced therapies such as weight loss medications, weight loss devices, and weight loss procedures should not be performed without a foundation of diet, activity, and behavior education and support, which should continue after the initiation of the advanced therapeutic modalities. Obesity should be approached as a chronic, incurable disease.

Healthy living practices should be applied to the whole family unit and supported by the school and community.[17,18] Consistency in the child's environment is essential. The adoption of healthy living activities is beneficial to all family members without regard to their individual weight status.

Which diet to advise is controversial. Even agreement on what is a healthy diet is difficult. Appreciating cultural and ethnic background is important to improve the acceptance and continuation of a healthy diet. Ketogenic diets, very-low-calorie diets, and meal replacement systems may be useful at the initiation of weight management, but eventually a healthy everyday diet should be attained, and this may involve considerable creativity on the part of the team's dietitian, depending on the cultural and ethnic background of the patient and family.

Dr Robert Lustig[19] observes: "Parents won't change until you show them:

1. Their kid will eat the food;
2. Other people's kids will eat the food;
3. They themselves like the food; and
4. They can afford the food."

Obesity is a heterogenous disease and there is variation in how different patients handle different caloric sources. The macronutrients and micronutrients need to be calculated to avoid starvation; achieve modulation to a healthy body composition; and support health, growth, and development.

Activity is important for health and for maintenance of a healthy body composition. It is not efficient or effective as a stand-alone therapeutic technique to attain a healthy body composition. Children with obesity frequently have orthopedic and mechanical difficulties in performing the usual activities for their age. Because of the difficulties children with obesity can have with certain activities, a physical therapist should be part of the weight management team. The activity portion of healthy living has to be fun, safe, and available. Current activity guidelines use time and level of exertion as markers. Time is difficult because of the spontaneous nature of activity in children.

Level of exertion is highly subjective without complex monitoring. Evaluation and monitoring of the fitness level of children with obesity can be done with the Harvard Step Test,[20] the 6-minute walk/run,[21] or the Bruce Protocol,[22] although these are not designed for children with obesity.

BARIATRIC SURGICAL PROCEDURES

Reports over the last 20 to 25 years have established that bariatric surgical procedures can be safely and effectively performed in children and adolescents with obesity.[23–26] Unique concerns about children and adolescents with obesity being treated with bariatric surgical procedures have included:

1. Would weight management with surgical procedures cause problems with growth and development?
2. Would children, adolescents, and families be able to adapt to the dietary and behavioral requirements before and after a bariatric surgical procedure?
3. Would weight management with surgical procedures for children, adolescents, and families result in resolution or prevention of the medical and psychosocial comorbidities of obesity?
4. Would the risks and complications of bariatric surgical procedures be balanced out by the improvements in quality of life and resolution or prevention of the medical and psychosocial comorbidities of obesity?
5. Would the cost of bariatric surgical procedures, including ensuing complications and revisions, be balanced out by the improved economic productivity of children or adolescents with obesity as they move on into adulthood?

The most common bariatric surgical procedures currently being performed for weight management of children and adolescents with obesity include the laparoscopic sleeve gastrectomy (LSG), the Roux-en-Y gastric bypass (RYGB), and the adjustable gastric band (AGB).[27] There has been a small, published experience with the biliopancreatic diversion and duodenal switch, but possible nutritional consequences have steered surgeons away from using these procedures for weight management in children and adolescents.

The longest experience in the pediatric population has been with the RYGB, which is usually performed laparoscopically. When performing the RYGB, the surgeon creates a small proximal gastric pouch attached to a Roux-en-Y limb of jejunum, resulting in bypass of the mid and distal stomach, the duodenum, and the proximal part of the jejunum. RYGB was originally thought to be effective because of the restriction caused by the small proximal gastric pouch and because of malabsorption caused by the bypass of portions of the stomach, the duodenum, and the proximal jejunum. Newer understanding of the energy regulatory system, including the importance of the vagus nerve and hormones secreted by the stomach, duodenum, and small intestine, shows that most of the RYGB effects are physiologic. These effects include stimulation of afferent signals from the stomach to the hypothalamus via the vagus nerve, and the altered stimulation of hormones secreted by the duodenum, jejunum, and ileum.[28,29] There is a bell-shaped curve to the responses to the RYGB with nonresponders and super-responders. The average response is about a 50% to 60% excess weight loss over the first 6 to 12 months after the procedure with good maintenance of a healthier body composition for at least 3 years.[26]

Five to 10 years ago, there was considerable experience using the AGB for weight management of obese adolescents.[30–35] The AGB is an adjustable silicon ring placed around the upper stomach to create a small proximal gastric pouch. The mechanism for weight loss is decreased hunger mediated by the vagus nerve responding to the pressure in the small proximal gastric pouch. Adjustment of the ring size is achieved by injecting or removing fluid from a balloon on the inner surface of the ring. The average response is about 40% to 50% excess weight loss over 3 years. There is little response immediately after placement of the AGB. Response depends on the AGB being adjusted to the point at which the patient's hunger is resolved with a small portion of food. This point seems to depend on the size of the orifice through the ring, which changes in response to the thinning or thickening of the stomach passing through the ring. Therefore, repeated adjustments are often necessary. The AGB requires continued management by a weight management program to support the mechanical nature of the patient's diet, the necessary adjustments of the AGB, and the potential management of food impaction and proximal pouch dilatation. Several factors have resulted in decreased use of this modality in the United States, including slower or minimal response to therapy, and the need for long-term management of the patient.

The newest weight loss procedure is the LSG, which involves the removal of 80% to 90% of the stomach by resecting longitudinally along the lesser curve and creating a tubular stomach. The procedure results in signals to the ERS by several mechanisms: (1) pressure in the proximal stomach; (2) reduction of ghrelin production through removal of most of the ghrelin-producing cells in the stomach; and (3) shortened gastric emptying time, resulting in faster stimulation of the distal small bowel and leading to increased levels or peptide YY (PYY) and glucagon-like peptide-1 (GLP-1) (satiety signaling mechanism). The weight loss with LSG is approximately 50% of excess weight loss and occurs over the first year after the operation. The simplicity, safety, and effectiveness of the LSG has resulted in it becoming the most common weight loss procedure performed in the United States.[36]

At present, the responses to the previous unique concerns regarding children and adolescents and bariatric surgical procedures are as follows:

1. Would weight management with surgical procedures cause problems with growth and development? There has been no evidence that weight management with surgical procedures causes problems with growth and development.[37] Weight management with surgical procedures usually results in a healthier body composition but does not result in a normal body composition, underweight, or malnutrition.
2. Would the children, adolescents, and families be able to adapt to the dietary and behavioral requirements before and after a bariatric surgical procedure? All the published experience has shown that the results from weight management with surgical procedures for children and adolescents with obesity is at least as good as the results in adults and does not produce any unique complications.
3. Would weight management with surgical procedures for children, adolescents, and families result in resolution or prevention of the medical and psychosocial comorbidities of obesity? The early results are encouraging, but there are no large, long-term studies.
4. Would the risks and complications of bariatric surgical procedures be balanced out by improvements in quality of life and resolution or prevention of the medical and psychosocial comorbidities of obesity? The early results are encouraging, but there are no large, long-term studies.
5. Would the cost of bariatric surgical procedures, including ensuing complications and revisions, be balanced out by the improved economic productivity of children or adolescents with obesity as they move on into adulthood? The authors currently do not know the answer. This question will require long-term, comprehensive studies.

In spite of the answers to these concerns, support for weight management with bariatric surgical procedures for children and adolescents with obesity from clinicians, policy makers, and payers has been slow to develop. In the adult world, the use of weight management with bariatric surgery occurs in less than 1% of the candidates. The limited use of bariatric surgical therapy has created a gap between healthy living techniques to treat obesity and the use of bariatric surgery. Obese adults who fail to adequately respond to managing their obesity with healthy living are offered pharmacotherapy, weight loss devices, and bariatric surgery. The treatment gap is wider for children and adolescents because of the greater reluctance to use bariatric surgery, even more limited pharmacotherapy options, and the lack of other options. In addition, the decision-making process for obese children and adolescents is more complicated than for adults because it involves their parents and their primary care physicians. The recent advent of safe, effective, US Food and Drug Administration (FDA)–approved devices for obese adults has the potential to fill the gap between healthy living techniques and bariatric surgery. Additional studies investigating the safety and efficacy of weight loss medications and devices in children and adolescents are needed.

WEIGHT LOSS MEDICATIONS

Obesity is a physiologic dysfunction of the energy regulatory system in susceptible people in the modern environment. High-sugar diets lead to increased serum insulin levels and insulin blocks leptin at the hypothalamus. Some macronutrients (fructose) are used to make fat and are not used for energy. Lack of fiber changes the glycemic index and slows the stimulation of the intestine to produce GLP-1. In susceptible people, the energy management system goes awry in the current environment. The energy management system defends an unhealthy body composition. In response to attempts to lose weight or change the body composition to a more healthy state, hunger and slower metabolism block the attempt at attaining a healthy body composition.

Weight loss medications act on the gastrointestinal (GI) tract, in the central nervous system, or both. They can be temporary and they can be titrated. They may be uniquely suited for use in children because obese children may be at a more plastic phase in the disease of obesity. If the children can achieve a healthy body composition, they may be able to sustain that healthy body composition with healthy living techniques; a process most adults cannot achieve. However, the use of weight loss medications in children and adolescents with obesity is complicated by issues around FDA approval for this population. With the current paradigm of FDA medication approval, it takes an average of 10 years for a medication to go from approval for use in adults to approval for use in children. Most of the medications currently non–FDA approved for weight management have been used in children for other indications (topiramate for seizures, bupropion for depression, naltrexone for smoking cessation and opioid addiction, metformin for type 2 diabetes and polycystic ovary syndrome, lisdexamfetamine for binge-eating disorders, and levoamphetamine/dextroamphetamine for attention-deficit/hyperactivity disorder) and weight loss has been noted as a side effect (**Table 3**).

Many medications may be useful to treat children with obesity. Given the complexity of the energy regulatory system and the heterogeneity of the response to each medication, there are many possibilities to be explored. One pathway is to work out phenotypes, genotypes, and biochemical profiles to predict which patient will have a better response to a particular medication. Future studies should explore (1) the use of pharmacotherapy before and after bariatric surgical procedures, (2) the possibility

Table 3
Weight loss medications

Generic Name	Trade Names	Mechanisms of Action	FDA Approved for Weight Loss
Orlistat	Xenical, Alli	Blocks fat absorption in GI tract	Yes, down to age 12 y
Phentermine	Adipex-P, Suprenza	Norepinephrine reuptake inhibition	Yes, down to age 17 y
Topiramate	Topamax	Modulation of GABA	No
Bupropion	Wellbutrin	Epinephrine and norepinephrine reuptake inhibition	No
Naltrexone	Revia	Opioid receptor antagonism	No
Metformin	Glucophage	Activation of adenosine monophosphate activated protein kinase	No
Lisdexamfetamine	Vyvanse	Norepinephrine and dopamine reuptake inhibition	No
Levoamphetamine and dextroamphetamine	Adderall	Norepinephrine and dopamine reuptake inhibition	No
Lorcaserin	Belviq	Selective serotonin 5-hydroxytryptamine receptor 2C (5-HT2C) receptor agonist	Yes, down to age 18 y
Eventide	Byetta	GLP-1 agonist	No
Liraglutide	Saxenda	GLP-1 agonist	Yes, down to age 18 y
Phentermine plus topiramate	Qsymia	Norepinephrine reuptake inhibition plus modulation of GABA	Yes, down to age 18 y
Bupropion plus naltrexone	Contrave	Epinephrine and norepinephrine reuptake inhibition plus opioid receptor antagonism	Yes, down to age 18 y

Abbreviation: GABA, gamma-aminobutyric acid.

of combination therapy using multiple medications either synchronously or metachronously, and (3) combining pharmacotherapy with weight loss devices.

WEIGHT LOSS DEVICES

Weight loss devices can be characterized by removability and adjustability. Some are mechanical and some are physiologic. Some are temporary and some are permanent. Their use is controversial for the same reasons weight loss medications are controversial. Note that their flexibility may make them more suited for obese pediatric patients, especially if the child is able to attain and maintain a healthy body composition with the aid of healthy living and weight loss devices, weight loss medications, or a combination of weight loss devices and medications. As with all other advanced techniques for weight management, a foundation of healthy living (diet, activity, and behavior) is essential. This foundation needs to be established before using an advanced technique and continued thereafter.

There are more than 20 weight loss devices commercially available worldwide (**Tables 4–8**). Four weight loss devices are currently FDA approved for use in weight management of adults with obesity: single gastric balloon, double gastric balloon,

Table 4
Weight loss devices: intragastric

Name	Placement	FDA Approved	Adjustable
Orbera	Endoscopic	Yes	No
Reshape Duo-Balloon	Endoscopic	Yes	No
Spatz	Endoscopic	No	Yes
Heliosphere	Endoscopic	No	No
Endogast	Endoscopic	No	Yes
Obalon	Swallowed	No	No
Ellipse	Swallowed	No	Yes
Transpyloric shuttle	Endoscopic	No	No
Gellesis 100	Swallowed	No	Yes

Table 5
Weight loss devices: extragastric

Name	Placement	FDA Approved	Adjustable
Lap-band	Laparoscopic	Yes	Yes
Realize band	Laparoscopic	Yes	Yes
Midband	Laparoscopic	No	Yes
Heliogast	Laparoscopic	No	Yes
Bioring	Laparoscopic	No	Yes
Prevail	Laparoscopic	No	Yes
Gastric Vest	Laparoscopic	No	No

Table 6
Weight loss devices: neuromodulation

Name	Placement	FDA Approved	Adjustable
Maestro: VBLOC	Laparoscopic	Yes	Yes
Abiliti	Laparoscopic	No	Yes
Diamond	Laparoscopic	No	Yes

Table 7
Weight loss devices: duodenal

Name	Placement	FDA Approved	Adjustable
EndoBarrier	Endoscopic	No	No
SatiSphere	Endoscopic	No	No
Revita	Endoscopic	No	No
MetaboShield	Endoscopic	No	No

Abbreviation: DMR, duodenal mucosal resurfacing.

Table 8 Weight loss devices: others			
Name	Placement	FDA Approved	Adjustable
Small Bite	Dentist	No	Yes
Aspire: gastric drainage	Endoscopic	Yes	Yes

vagal stimulation device, and gastric drainage device. At present, none of the weight loss devices are FDA approved for use in obese individuals less than 18 years of age. The question is what characteristics and mechanisms of action might be optimal in children with obesity.

Laparoscopically placed devices, such as the vagal stimulator, the gastric stimulator, the AGB, and the perigastric vest, are not ideal because of the invasive nature of placement. They are adjustable, removable, and designed to be permanent.

Devices such as the intragastric balloons, the transpyloric shuttle, the duodenal balloons, the gastroduodenal sleeve, and the duodenal-jejunal sleeve involve upper endoscopy for placement. Some new balloons under study are designed to be swallowed. One of these automatically deflates and is passed spontaneously, thus avoiding any need for endoscopy to remove it. The standard and approved balloons are removed with a second endoscopy, as are the shuttle and sleeves.

Some of the intragastric balloons are adjustable; one with repeat endoscopy and one via a transabdominal catheter attached to a subcutaneous port. However, multiple small intragastric balloons can be placed sequentially. Adjustability may help with the initial tolerance of the intragastric balloons, which is a potential problem with children. The transpyloric shuttle, the duodenal balloons, and the sleeves are not adjustable.

One unique device is multiple hydrogel particles packed into a capsule. The capsule is swallowed before a meal, and the hydrogel beads swell with the liquid in the stomach, slow gastric emptying, create gastric fullness, and retard glucose absorption in the small intestine. They then dehydrate in the colon and are passed spontaneously.

Another weight loss methodology is the recently approved gastric drainage device. A percutaneous endoscopic gastrostomy is placed with a special attachment to connect intermittently to an aspiration system. After eating, the patients drain a portion of their gastric contents and discard it. This device is recently FDA approved for use in adults and weight loss results are reasonable. Remarkably, there has been good acceptance in selected patients and no fluid or electrolyte abnormalities have been discovered.

Many weight loss devices may be useful to treat children with obesity. Given the uniqueness of children, the complexity of the energy regulatory system, and the heterogeneity of the response to each device, there are many possibilities to be explored. As for weight loss medications, analyzing phenotypes, genotypes, and biochemical profiles to predict which patients will have a better response to a particular device would be ideal. Future studies need to explore the (1) safety and efficacy of endoscopically placed weight loss devices in the pediatric population, (2) placement timing and duration of temporary devices, and (3) use of endoscopic devices in conjunction with pharmacotherapy or as a bridge to surgical weight loss procedures.

ENDOSCOPIC WEIGHT LOSS PROCEDURES

Endoscopic weight loss procedures are performed with laparoscopes and/or GI endoscopes, mimic many of the surgical bariatric procedures, and do not involve resection of tissue (**Table 9**). A narrowing of the stomach can be produced near the

Table 9
Endoscopic weight loss procedures

Procedure	Mimic
TERIS procedure	Gastric band
1. Laparoscopic gastric plication 2. Gastroscopic gastric plication	Sleeve gastrectomy
NOTES procedure	RYGB

Abbreviations: NOTES, natural orifice transluminal endoscopic surgery; TERIS, Transoral Endoscopic Restrictive Implant System.

gastroesophageal junction, mimicking an AGB, while working transorally with a gastroscope. Endoscopically, the volume of the stomach can be reduced, mimicking a gastric sleeve resection, working transorally or working with a laparoscopic approach. Endoscopically a bypass of the distal stomach to the jejunum can even be produced, mimicking an RYGB. These approaches are attractive because they may make weight loss procedures more acceptable to patients and their families. They are perceived as less invasive, they may involve sedation rather than general anesthesia, they may involve shorter time in the hospital, and they may allow a faster return to regular diet and activities. These procedures may help fill the gap between healthy living techniques and bariatric surgical procedures. Any of these advantages would apply to children and adolescents with obesity just as they do to adults with obesity.

The basic challenges to these procedures are instrumentation and durability. The instrumentation is advancing rapidly with trials already published of both gastric[38,39] and laparoscopic[40,41] imbrication of the stomach mimicking a gastric sleeve resection and of gastroscopic narrowing of the proximal stomach to create a small proximal gastric pouch mimicking an AGB.[42] There has also been pilot work done on using a gastroscopic approach to work transorally, exit the stomach inside out, identify the proximal jejunum, and anastomose the jejunum to the stomach to create a gastrojejunal bypass.[43] The short-term results are fair and the procedures are safe. However, durability remains a problem and safe, more durable tissue fixation techniques need to be developed.

OTHER TECHNIQUES

As the physiology of obesity is better understood and the multiple factors involved are discovered, more imaginative, safer, less invasive, and more adjustable techniques of weight management are being explored. The microbiome in the GI tract is one of these areas. Variations in the microbiome between patients with obesity and patients without obesity are being identified. Mechanisms by which the microbiome affects the energy regulatory system are being discovered. Experiments in laboratory animals have shown the ability to cause obesity by transferring the microbiome from an obese laboratory animal to a lean laboratory animal. The effects of antibiotics and other commonly used drugs, such as those used for gastroesophageal reflux disease, on the microbiome are being studied. Clinicians are defining the anatomic areas in the brain that are involved in the energy management system, and transcranial stimulation techniques to specific areas of the brain are being developed.

SUMMARY

The obesity epidemic in the pediatric population has serious clinical and psychosocial consequences, including effects on health, quality of life, economic productivity, and consumption of health care resources during childhood and adulthood. The basics of weight management in children and adolescents are healthy living techniques with diet, activity, and behavior. The physiology of obesity blocks these efforts in many children and adolescents and additional methods are needed to control the disease. Bariatric surgery procedures are safe and effective but they are not typically acceptable, applicable, and available to many children and adolescents. Weight loss medications and weight loss devices are available, but most of them are not FDA approved for use in children and adolescents. However, these techniques may be uniquely suited to the obese pediatric population. Endoscopic bariatric procedures offer considerable promise to children and adolescents with obesity, but the issue of durability needs to be conquered.

Prevention is ultimately the best method to solve the problem of obesity in children and adolescents; in the meantime, obese children need safe, effective, available treatment. In the near future, GI endoscopists will be key to weight management programs for children and adolescents with obesity.

REFERENCES

1. Sonntag D, Ali S, Lehnert T, et al. Estimating the lifetime cost of childhood obesity in Germany: results of a Markov model. Pediatr Obes 2015;10(6):416–22.
2. Sonntag D, Ali S, De Bock F. Lifetime indirect cost of childhood overweight and obesity: a decision analytic model. Obesity (Silver Spring) 2016;24(1):200–6.
3. Ben-David K, Rossidis G. Bariatric surgery: indications, safety and efficacy. Curr Pharm Des 2011;17(12):1209–17.
4. Ginsberg GM, Rosenberg E. Economic effects of interventions to reduce obesity in Israel. Isr J Health Policy Res 2012;1(1):17.
5. Fonvig CE, Chabanova E, Ohrt JD, et al. Multidisciplinary care of obese children and adolescents for one year reduces ectopic fat content in liver and skeletal muscle. BMC Pediatr 2015;15:196.
6. Foster BA, Farragher J, Parker P, et al. Treatment interventions for early childhood obesity: a systematic review. Acad Pediatr 2015;15(4):353–61.
7. Gurnani M, Birken C, Hamilton J. Childhood obesity: causes, consequences, and management. Pediatr Clin North Am 2015;62(4):821–40.
8. CDC. Individual Growth Charts. 2009. Available at: http://www.cdc.gov/growthcharts/charts.htm. Accessed January 25, 2017.
9. Skinner AC, Perrin EM, Skelton JA. Prevalence of obesity and severe obesity in US children, 1999-2014. Obesity (Silver Spring) 2016;24(5):1116–23.
10. Varni JW. PedsQ. Available at: http://www.pedsql.org/about_pedsql.html. Accessed January 25, 2017.
11. Puhl RM, King KM. Weight discrimination and bullying. Best Pract Res Clin Endocrinol Metab 2013;27(2):117–27.
12. Barlow SE, Expert C. Expert committee recommendations regarding the prevention, assessment, and treatment of child and adolescent overweight and obesity: summary report. Pediatrics 2007;120(Suppl 4):S164–92.
13. Whitlock EP, Williams SB, Gold R, et al. Screening and interventions for childhood overweight: a summary of evidence for the US Preventive Services Task Force. Pediatrics 2005;116(1):e125–44.
14. Epstein LH, Paluch RA, Roemmich JN, et al. Family-based obesity treatment, then and now: twenty-five years of pediatric obesity treatment. Health Psychol 2007;26(4):381–91.

15. McGovern L, Johnson JN, Paulo R, et al. Clinical review: treatment of pediatric obesity: a systematic review and meta-analysis of randomized trials. J Clin Endocrinol Metab 2008;93(12):4600–5.
16. Ho M, Garnett SP, Baur L, et al. Effectiveness of lifestyle interventions in child obesity: systematic review with meta-analysis. Pediatrics 2012;130(6):e1647–71.
17. Rogers VW, Hart PH, Motyka E, et al. Impact of Let's Go! 5-2-1-0: a community-based, multisetting childhood obesity prevention program. J Pediatr Psychol 2013;38(9):1010–20.
18. Kessler HL, Vine J, Rogers VW. Let's go! school nutrition workgroups: regional partnerships for improving school meals. J Nutr Educ Behav 2015;47(3):278–82.
19. Lustig RH, Millar H, Gershen C. The fat chance cookbook: more than 100 recipes ready in under 30 minutes to help you lose the sugar and the weight. New York: Hudson Street Press; 2013.
20. Sloan AW. The Harvard step test of dynamic fitness. Triangle 1962;5:358–63.
21. Pereira AC, Ribeiro MG, Araujo AP. Timed motor function tests capacity in healthy children. Arch Dis Child 2016;101(2):147–51.
22. van der Cammen-van Zijp MH, Ijsselstijn H, Takken T, et al. Exercise testing of pre-school children using the Bruce treadmill protocol: new reference values. Eur J Appl Physiol 2010;108(2):393–9.
23. Breaux CW. Obesity surgery in children. Obes Surg 1995;5(3):279–84.
24. Treadwell JR, Sun F, Schoelles K. Systematic review and meta-analysis of bariatric surgery for pediatric obesity. Ann Surg 2008;248(5):763–76.
25. Cozacov Y, Roy M, Moon S, et al. Mid-term results of laparoscopic sleeve gastrectomy and Roux-en-Y gastric bypass in adolescent patients. Obes Surg 2014;24(5):747–52.
26. Inge TH, Courcoulas AP, Jenkins TM, et al. Weight loss and health status 3 years after bariatric surgery in adolescents. N Engl J Med 2016;374(2):113–23.
27. Zwintscher NP, Azarow KS, Horton JD, et al. The increasing incidence of adolescent bariatric surgery. J Pediatr Surg 2013;48(12):2401–7.
28. Lutz TA, Bueter M. Physiological mechanisms behind Roux-en-Y gastric bypass surgery. Dig Surg 2014;31(1):13–24.
29. Abdeen G, le Roux CW. Mechanism underlying the weight loss and complications of Roux-en-Y gastric bypass [review]. Obes Surg 2016;26(2):410–21.
30. Loy JJ, Youn HA, Schwack B, et al. Improvement in nonalcoholic fatty liver disease and metabolic syndrome in adolescents undergoing bariatric surgery. Surg Obes Relat Dis 2015;11(2):442–9.
31. Holterman AX, Browne A, Dillard BE 3rd, et al. Short-term outcome in the first 10 morbidly obese adolescent patients in the FDA-approved trial for laparoscopic adjustable gastric banding. J Pediatr Gastroenterol Nutr 2007;45(4):465–73.
32. Nadler EP, Youn HA, Ren CJ, et al. An update on 73 US obese pediatric patients treated with laparoscopic adjustable gastric banding: comorbidity resolution and compliance data. J Pediatr Surg 2008;43(1):141–6.
33. Black JA, White B, Viner RM, et al. Bariatric surgery for obese children and adolescents: a systematic review and meta-analysis. Obes Rev 2013;14(8):634–44.
34. Messiah SE, Lopez-Mitnik G, Winegar D, et al. Changes in weight and co-morbidities among adolescents undergoing bariatric surgery: 1-year results from the Bariatric Outcomes Longitudinal Database. Surg Obes Relat Dis 2013; 9(4):503–13.
35. Jelin EB, Daggag H, Speer AL, et al. Melanocortin-4 receptor signaling is not required for short-term weight loss after sleeve gastrectomy in pediatric patients. Int J Obes (Lond) 2016;40(3):550–3.

36. Ponce J, Nguyen NT, Hutter M, et al. American Society for metabolic and bariatric surgery estimation of bariatric surgery procedures in the United States, 2011-2014. Surg Obes Relat Dis 2015;11(6):1199–200.

37. Alqahtani A, Elahmedi M, Qahtani AR. Laparoscopic sleeve gastrectomy in children younger than 14 years: refuting the concerns. Ann Surg 2016;263(2): 312–9.

38. Verlaan T, Paulus GF, Mathus-Vliegen EM, et al. Endoscopic gastric volume reduction with a novel articulating plication device is safe and effective in the treatment of obesity (with video). Gastrointest Endosc 2015;81(2):312–20.

39. Lopez-Nava Breviere G, Bautista-Castano I, Fernandez-Corbelle JP, et al. Endoscopic sleeve gastroplasty (the Apollo method): a new approach to obesity management. Rev Esp Enferm Dig 2016;108(4):201–6.

40. Albanese A, Prevedello L, Verdi D, et al. Laparoscopic gastric plication: an emerging bariatric procedure with high surgical revision rate. Bariatr Surg Pract Patient Care 2015;10(3):93–8.

41. Chouillard E, Schoucair N, Alsabah S, et al. Laparoscopic gastric plication (LGP) as an alternative to laparoscopic sleeve gastrectomy (LSG) in patients with morbid obesity: a preliminary, short-term, case-control study. Obes Surg 2016; 26(6):1167–72.

42. Verlaan T, de Jong K, de la Mar-Ploem ED, et al. Trans-oral endoscopic restrictive implant system: endoscopic treatment of obesity? Surg Obes Relat Dis 2016; 12(9):1711–8.

43. Kumar N. Weight loss endoscopy: development, applications, and current status. World J Gastroenterol 2016;22(31):7069–79.

The Regulatory Perspectives on Endoscopic Devices for Obesity

April K. Marrone, PhD, MBA*, Mark J. Antonino, MS,
Joshua S. Silverstein, PhD, Martha W. Betz, PhD,
Priya Venkataraman-Rao, MD, Martin Golding, MD,
Diane Cordray, VMD, Jeffrey W. Cooper, DVM

KEYWORDS

- Obesity • Medical device • Regulatory • Intragastric balloon • Gastric emptying
- Endoscopic • Weight loss

KEY POINTS

- There are 3 major pathways to legally market a device: premarket notification (510[k]), premarket approval, and de novo classification.
- The US Food and Drug Administration (FDA) principally relies on nonclinical and clinical studies to assess device benefits and risks.
- FDA-approved endoscopic weight-loss devices to date include the 3 intragastric balloons, ReShape, ORBERA, and Obalon, and the gastric-emptying device, the AspireAssist.
- The FDA has a published benefit-risk paradigm to aid in the development of clinical studies.
- The Patient Preference Calculator for Weight-Loss Devices indicates that 6% to 7% of patients consider a device with a profile similar to intragastric balloons to be better than no device, considering 6-month weight loss benefits; 11% to 22% consider a device with a profile similar to gastric-emptying devices to be better than no device considering the 12-month weight-loss benefit.

INTRODUCTION

Obesity is a chronic, relapsing health risk defined by excess body fat. Excessive body fat increases the risk of death and major comorbidities, such as type 2 diabetes, hypertension, dyslipidemia, cardiovascular disease, sleep apnea, osteoarthritis, asthma, back pain, and some cancers.[1,2] Current treatment options for individuals with obesity

Disclosure Statement: The authors have nothing to disclose.
Gastroenterology Devices Branch of the Division of Reproductive Gastro-Renal and Urological Devices, Center for Devices and Radiological Health, U.S. Food and Drug Administration, 10903 New Hampshire Avenue, Building 66, Room G218, Silver Spring, MD 20993-0002, USA
* Corresponding author.
E-mail address: April.Marrone@fda.hhs.gov

Gastrointest Endoscopy Clin N Am 27 (2017) 327–341
http://dx.doi.org/10.1016/j.giec.2016.12.004
1052-5157/17/Published by Elsevier Inc.

giendo.theclinics.com

range from diet and exercise with and without behavior modification to the higher-risk option of bariatric surgery. Pharmacotherapies are potential options for individuals who have failed to respond to lifestyle interventions and are either not able or willing to undergo bariatric surgery.

Drugs intended for weight loss or weight management are reviewed through the US Food and Drug Administration (FDA) Center for Drug Evaluation and Research (CDER). Currently, CDER has approved orlistat, lorcaserin, phentermine/topiramate, naltrexone/bupropion, and liraglutide.[3–7] Surgical options include the Roux-en-Y gastric bypass (RYGB), sleeve gastrectomy, and biliopancreatic diversion with duodenal switch. The RYGB procedure results in most of the stomach and duodenum being bypassed. Vertical sleeve gastrectomy permanently reduces the size of the stomach, whereas the biliopancreatic diversion with duodenal switch results in most of the small intestine being bypassed.

Medical devices used for weight loss are regulated in the FDA Center for Devices and Radiological Health (CDRH) and are reviewed by the Gastroenterology Devices Branch (GEDB) in the Division of Reproductive Gastro-Renal and Urological Devices (DRGUD). In general, the weight-loss-device landscape can be divided into 6 main categories: (1) restrictive procedures, (2) space-occupying, (3) bypass liners, (4) electrical stimulation, (5) gastric emptying, and (6) other therapies. CDRH has approved 2 restrictive devices: the LAP-BAND Adjustable Band and the REALIZE Adjustable Band.[8,9] Currently, there is mention of restrictive procedures carried out using endoscopic suturing devices.[10,11] To date, there are no endoscopic suturing devices with marketing authorization for obesity indications. Although the first device approved by the FDA for weight loss was a space-occupying device, the Garren Gastric Bubble in 1985, it was later voluntarily removed from the market due to safety concerns. The FDA did not approve any further space-occupying devices until the ReShape, ORBERA, and Obalon intragastric balloons (IGBs) in 2015 to 2016.[12–14] The laparoscopically placed MAESTRO Rechargeable System has also received FDA approval in 2015 with the mechanism of action of delivering electrical signals to the vagus nerve.[15] In 2016, the FDA approved the AspireAssist device that partially empties stomach contents 20 to 30 minutes after eating.[16] Currently, the FDA has not approved a bypass liner for weight loss. However, the FDA is aware that bypass liners and other weight-loss devices are available outside of the United States and/or are currently in clinical testing.[11,17,18]

The number and type of device-treatment options available globally, and specifically in the United States, demonstrate that more choices for obesity treatment are being developed to meet the needs of the patient population. Although reduction of excessive body fat may reduce the risks of obesity-associated comorbidities, such as metabolic disorders, at this time no device has been approved for use in the United States that is indicated for treatment of metabolic disorders.

Of the FDA-approved weight-loss devices, those placed endoscopically include the space-occupying IGBs and the gastric-emptying device. The FDA considers both the benefits and the risks associated with the device during the review process. Here, the clinical trial development, regulatory pathways, and considerations used during FDA review of weight-loss devices, and the benefit-risk analysis of the recently FDA-approved endoscopic weight-loss devices, are discussed. In addition, a strategic priority of CDRH is to increase patient input in decision making,[19] and CDRH previously developed a data-derived tool that estimates patient preference for obesity-treatment devices.[20] Thus, how devices with profiles similar to those that have been recently approved may be viewed in light of the patient preference study also is considered.[20,21]

DISCUSSION
Regulatory Pathways for Obesity Devices

Medical devices are classified into 3 groups: class I, II, and III. Class I devices are considered to be low risk, whereas class III devices have the highest risk. There are 3 major pathways to legally market a device: premarket notification (510[k]), premarket approval (PMA), and de novo classification. Clinical data are generally necessary to support de novo or PMA applications. Approximately 10% of 510(k)s require clinical data. For investigational devices, clinical data are collected for significant risk studies in the United States under an Investigational Device Exemption (IDE).

Premarket notification (510[k])

For medical devices subject to premarket notification, a 510(k) must be submitted.[22] The device is compared with a predicate, which is a previously 510(k)-cleared device, a device granted marketing authorization via a de novo classification request, or a device marketed before the 1976 Medical Device Amendments. The 510(k) should demonstrate that a device is at least as safe and as effective as a legally marketed predicate device through comparison of the intended use and technological characteristics. Any differences in the indications for use or technological characteristics and whether these differences alter safety and effectiveness should be discussed and, as necessary, supported by performance data. A device determined to be substantially equivalent (SE) to the predicate can be legally marketed. Extensive information regarding the 510(k) process is available.[23] Currently, there are no devices with specific obesity indications that have been cleared through the 510(k) process.

The de novo classification process

For devices that do not fall within an existing classification regulation, but present low or moderate risk, a de novo request may be appropriate. Briefly, a device should be able to demonstrate a reasonable assurance of safety and effectiveness (RASE) through the use of general and/or special controls.[24] Special controls may include nonclinical or clinical testing, and labeling requirements. The FDA will make a benefit-risk determination for the device during de novo review.[25] If the data demonstrate RASE with appropriate risk mitigation, the de novo can be granted and allow for marketing authorization of the medical device. Granting a de novo request creates a new classification regulation, and the device can serve as a predicate for future devices through the 510(k) process. Currently, there are no endoscopic devices with specific weight-loss indications for which requests for de novo classification have been granted.

The premarket approval process

A PMA application is typically necessary for class III devices, where general and special controls are insufficient to provide RASE. These devices support or sustain human life, are of substantial importance in preventing impairment of human health, or present a potential, unreasonable risk of illness or injury.[26,27] A PMA application typically includes summaries and detailed reports of nonclinical and clinical testing, manufacturing information, and complete device labeling.

A PMA is reviewed to ensure that valid scientific evidence has been provided to support a determination of an RASE for the device's intended use. The FDA may refer a PMA to an advisory committee for review.[28] If the PMA is approved, the FDA imposes postapproval requirements, as necessary, which may include continuing evaluation of the safety, effectiveness, and reliability of the device. Currently, all obesity devices with a weight-loss indication have required a PMA application and postapproval studies.

Clinical Studies to Support Safety and Effectiveness of Obesity Treatment Devices

The IDE is the first formal step in conducting significant risk studies of investigational devices before device marketing.[29] Study sponsors develop the clinical trial design, statistical plan, and follow-up procedures needed to support future marketing applications. Effectiveness endpoints often include a hypothesis with a prespecified superiority margin for weight loss and a performance goal for a responder rate. Participants included in IDE obesity studies often have a body mass index (BMI) greater than 30 kg/m^2 and at least one obesity-related comorbidity. FDA may require specific monitoring plans or interim data analyses by independent data monitoring committees to ensure the safety of enrolled participants. The FDA encourages sponsors to review IDE guidance documents before submitting their IDE applications.[30,31]

Nonclinical testing

Nonclinical testing is usually necessary before initiation of a human study to assess device safety and performance. Typical nonclinical testing should demonstrate that the device is biocompatible and functions as intended through performance bench testing and possibly animal studies. The porcine model has been used most commonly to test obesity devices because porcine gastrointestinal anatomy and size are similar to human gastrointestinal anatomy and size.[12,32] However, pigs have several anatomic differences that should be considered in terms of device deployment and in vivo behavior, including a dorsal gastric shelf, more proximal esophageal and pyloric sphincters, and a longer, spiral colon.[33] Working within the limitations of the porcine model, animal studies can generate support for clinical safety particularly when the final device design is used and device delivery and use closely mimics clinical protocols.

Pediatric patients

Because the prevalence of children and adolescents with obesity has increased throughout the world,[34,35] and bariatric surgery carries potentially serious operative and perioperative complications, a medical device may present a viable option for some pediatric patients. However, the existing data are limited, and obtaining additional data has proven to be challenging given the lack of trials, ethical considerations, and concerns about whether the benefits would truly outweigh the risks in this vulnerable patient population. CDRH requests that special consideration be given to the design of clinical trials to support use of weight-loss devices in the pediatric population, which CDRH considers to be persons that are less than 22 years of age.[36]

The FDA convened the Pediatric Advisory Committee (PAC) in 2005 to discuss the clinical and ethical issues of pediatric obesity device trials.[37–39] The panel reached majority consensus on certain issues, including (1) the appropriate patient population (eg, eligibility criteria), (2) effectiveness and safety endpoints to measure, (3) trial designs, and (4) long-term safety and effectiveness issues and the role of postapproval studies. The panel made numerous recommendations, as follows:

- Devices, especially implants, should not be studied in the pediatric population until enough data have been gained from adult study and use.
- A staged introduction should be used when studying devices for obesity in the pediatric population.
- In general, long-term implant devices should be studied in patients with significant disease, which would be subjects in the 99th percentile for BMI for age and patients with at least one significant comorbidity.
- Study participants should be screened for known genetic causes of obesity and for Prader-Willi, and if included in the study, should be evaluated separately.

- Change in BMI would be an appropriate assessment tool for the primary effectiveness. For purposes of sample size calculation, a 5- to 7-point reduction in BMI would be a clinically meaningful reduction.
- Comorbidity reduction or resolution would be an important secondary effectiveness endpoint.
- A dissent clause should be included in the protocol.
- Provisions for reconsenting participants should be made as new data become available or as the children transition from assent to consent.
- Premarket data should be collected for 2 years, although participants should be consented/assented for 5 years.
- Studies should have a Data Monitoring Committee or Data Safety Monitoring Board.
- Studies should be done in centers where a multidisciplinary team with pediatric expertise is available, and dietary and behavior components of the study should be standardized between involved centers.
- Postapproval data should be collected through 5 years.
- Registries are encouraged.

The PAC's discussions are of use to device manufacturers who wish to pursue clinical studies to support a pediatric indication for obesity devices.

Benefit-risk paradigm

In a publication (ie, not a guidance document), the FDA has offered a benefit-risk paradigm for weight-loss devices meant to help study sponsors consider an appropriate effectiveness criteria for a pivotal study, based on safety data derived from a pilot study or other human experience with a device.[21] FDA's tiered approach was published following a public meeting in 2012 at which the Gastroenterology-Urology Devices Panel discussed benefits and risks of obesity devices.[40] Objective assessment criteria to be defined before initiation of a pivotal clinical study should consider important concepts of the benefit-risk assessment, such as the following[21,25]:

- Type of benefit
- Magnitude/duration of benefit
- Probability of a patient experiencing a benefit
- Number, severity, and type of harmful events associated with the use of the device
- Probability/duration of a harmful event

After information is gained from the pivotal study, the risks and benefits associated with the device can be re-evaluated.

Although there is no requirement to follow the paradigm, FDA offered 12 adverse event categories to characterize the levels of risk of devices, considering severity of the outcome.[21] Minimal-risk (level 1) devices may have high rates of the most mild events (eg, up to 100% experiencing discomfort that is addressed with over-the-counter medication), low rates of events of intermediate severity (eg, 2%–5% experiencing problems requiring prescription drugs), and very low rates of severe events (eg, <0.1% experiencing hospitalization). Increased rates of intermediate and severe events would be consistent with a level 2 risk categorization, whereas higher rates would be consistent with a level 3 or 4 risk categorization. According to the paradigm FDA offered, the overall risk for a device would be determined by the highest risk level for any adverse event category.

Effectiveness targets were also offered. CDER's expectations for weight-loss drugs, and the results obtained from the 2 weight-loss devices that had received FDA approval and were being marketed at the time of publication of the paradigm: the LAP-BAND and REALIZE banding devices, were considered.[8,9,41] The benefit scale considers the magnitude of the benefit, whether the benefit is relative to diet and exercise or sham procedure, the percentage of patients experiencing the benefit, and the time after device placement that the benefit is maintained.[21] Even though there are circumstances that make sham-controlled trials difficult, such as exposing patients to risk without benefit, and blinds that can be broken, shams do provide beneficial information regarding the true treatment effect offered by the device.

As new information is gained through use of emergent weight-loss-device therapies, the paradigm may be updated to better align with the evolving weight-loss-device landscape.

Benefit-Risk of US Food and Drug Administration–Approved Endoscopic Weight-Loss Devices

The FDA-approved endoscopic weight-loss medical devices are indicated for adults only and include the ReShape Integrated Dual Balloon System by ReShape Medical, Inc, San Clemente, CA (approved via P140012), the ORBERA Intragastric Balloon System by Apollo Endosurgery, Inc, Austin, TX (approved via P140008), the Obalon Balloon System by Obalon Therapeutics, Inc, Carlsbad, CA (approved via P160001), and the AspireAssist by Aspire Bariatric, Inc, King of Prussia, PA (approved via P150024).[12–14,16] The FDA has relied on clinical studies to assess device benefits and risks for endoscopic and other weight-loss devices. The quality of the clinical study design, the conduct of the study, the robustness of the study results, and the generalizability of results are taken into account. Assessments of benefit include addressing the type of benefit and evaluation of primary and secondary study effectiveness endpoints, including the percent total body weight loss (TBWL).[40] The magnitude and duration of the benefit are considered along with the probability of the patient experiencing one or more benefits.

In 2012, the FDA Obesity Device Panel did not provide a consensus recommendation for clinically meaningful weight loss.[40] FDA benefit considerations include weight loss measures proposed by CDER for drugs and the American Heart Association/American College of Cardiology/The Obesity Society 2013 prevention guideline.[41,42] As addressed in the 2013 prevention guideline, an initial weight loss goal of 5% to 10% within 6 months is recommended.[42,43] CDER Endocrinologic and Metabolic Drugs Advisory Committee meeting discussions for development of obesity drugs and CDER draft guidance for weight management drugs (draft guidance documents represent FDA's current thinking, but are not currently implemented) have recommended one of the following efficacy benchmarks after 1 year of treatment[41,44]:

- The difference in mean weight loss between the active-product and placebo-treated groups is at least 5% TBWL and the difference is statistically significant.
- The proportion of participants who lose 5% or more of baseline body weight in the active-product group is at least 35% and is approximately double the proportion in the placebo-treated group; the difference between groups is statistically significant.

The FDA considers whether the magnitude of benefit compensates for the means of achieving such a benefit. For instance, drug treatment can be stopped and explantable devices can be removed if complications arise. However, anatomic changes and permanently implanted devices are less readily reversed. Assessments of risk include an evaluation of device- or procedure-related serious adverse events (SAEs) and nonserious adverse events. The authors' assessment takes into account the probability and duration of harmful events, including the intervention required to address the harmful event. Where appropriate, risk mitigation, such as product labeling and establishing training programs, is also used to reduce or control risks.

Clinical studies performed to support FDA approval of endoscopic weight-loss devices have demonstrated observed %TBWL of 6.6% to 12.1% measured from 6 months to 1 year after device implantation (**Table 1**). Device- and procedure-related SAEs have varied from 0.3% to 10% for these endoscopic devices (see **Table 1**). **Fig. 1** shows %TBWL and SAE rates for FDA-approved weight-loss devices.

ReShape intragastric balloon
ReShape is a dual-balloon implant that consists of 2 independently saline-inflated, noncommunicating, 450-mL silicone balloons bonded to a central silicone shaft. The REDUCE clinical trial for the ReShape IGB was a randomized, double-blinded, sham-controlled study.[12] Participants randomized to the treatment group underwent a medically managed diet and exercise program for 48 weeks and had the ReShape IGB indwelling for 24 weeks. Control participants had a sham procedure and underwent the same diet and exercise program. At the end of the 24-week maximum balloon indwell treatment period, participants in the treatment arm experienced an average 6.8% TBWL (intent-to-treat population), whereas the participants in the sham-control arm of the study experienced an average of 3.3% TBWL (3.5% mean difference). At 48 weeks, treated participants who lost weight during the initial 24 weeks with the balloon had maintained a 4.8% TBWL. Ultimately, 49.4% of these participants maintained at least 40% of the weight lost at the time that ReShape was removed through the full 48-week study.

ORBERA intragastric balloon
ORBERA consists of a single 400- to 700-mL silicone elastomer balloon that is filled with saline and expands into a spherical shape. The IB-500 clinical trial for the ORBERA IGB was a randomized, nonblinded comparative study.[13] Participants randomized to the treatment group participated in a 12-month behavioral modification

---

Table 1
Average %TBWL as reported in the safety and effectiveness summaries for recently FDA-approved endoscopic weight-loss devices for treatment and control study subjects

Device	Study Arm	6 mo %TBWL	12 mo %TBWL	SAE Rate, %[a]
ReShape	Treatment	6.8[b]	4.8[b]	7.5
	Control	3.3	NA	NA
ORBERA	Treatment	10.2	7.6	10.0
	Control	3.3	3.1	NA
Obalon	Treatment	6.6[b]	5.7[b]	0.3
	Control	3.4	NA	NA
AspireAssist	Treatment	NA	12.1	3.6
	Control	NA	3.6	NA

SAE rate is procedure and/or device related and is from 6-month study data for the ReShape, ORBERA, and Obalon IGBs and 12-month study data for the AspireAssist gastric-emptying device.
Abbreviation: NA, not applicable.
  [a] The definition for an SAE is comparable across studies, for example, any adverse event resulting in death; any adverse event which is life-threatening; any adverse event resulting in hospitalization, or significant prolongation of an existing hospitalization; any adverse event resulting in a persistent, significant impairment; any adverse event requiring significant medical or surgical intervention to prevent a significant impairment; any adverse event resulting in a congenital anomaly or birth defect.
  [b] Data listed for 6 months are actually 24 weeks; data listed for 12 months are 48 weeks.

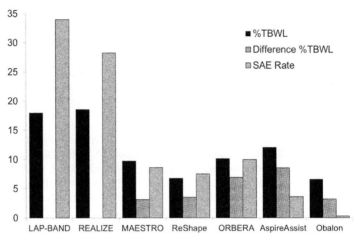

Fig. 1. %TBWL for clinical study treatment arms, difference between %TBWL for control and treatment arms, and %SAE rate reported in clinical studies used to support FDA approval of devices indicated for weight loss. The LAP-BAND and REALIZE gastric bands (approved via P000008 and P070009, respectively) used treatment participants as their own controls, and %TBWL is reported at 36 months after device placement. For the gastric bands, %TBWL was calculated by subtracting the baseline mean participant weight from the mean partici- pant weight at 36 months and then dividing by the mean baseline weight. The SAE rates are the percentage of study participants who reported at least one SAE that was procedure and/ or device related. LAP-BAND study participants reported severe adverse events at a rate of 34%, wherein serious and severe adverse events were most commonly addressed either by band adjustment or by reoperation to revise, replace, or remove either a component or the entire LAP-BAND System.[9] REALIZE participants (28.3%) reported 115 SAEs, of which 46 events were considered to not be related to the gastric band.[8] The MAESTRO device was approved via P130019, and the device labeling reports %TBWL for treatment and con- trol participants.[15,47] Details of the endoscopic weight-loss devices are discussed in the text.

program whereby the ORBERA IGB was indwelling for the first 6 months. Control participants were only in the behavioral modification program for 12 months. At the 6-month maximum balloon indwell treatment period, treatment participants (modified intent-to-treat population) experienced an average 10.2% TBWL, whereas control participants experienced an average 3.3% TBWL (6.9% mean difference). At the 12-month follow-up time point, treatment participants had maintained a 7.6% TBWL on average, whereas control participants had maintained a 3.1% TBWL (4.5% mean difference).

Obalon intragastric balloon (balloon system)
An Obalon balloon is introduced into the body by the participant swallowing a capsule attached to an inflation catheter. Once the capsule dissolves, the balloon is filled with gas. During the 24-week treatment period, a total of three 250-mL balloons can be placed into the participant's stomach. At the end of the treatment period, the balloons are removed endoscopically. The SMART clinical trial for the Obalon IGB was a pro- spective, sham-controlled, double-blinded, randomized comparative study.[14] Partic- ipants randomized to the treatment group received the Obalon Balloon System for 24 weeks and took part in a moderate-intensity diet and exercise program. Partici- pants in the control arm of the study received a sham capsule device without a balloon and took part in the behavioral modification program for 24 weeks. At the 24-week maximum treatment period, treatment participants experienced an average 6.6%

TBWL (modified intent-to-treat population), whereas control participants experienced an average 3.4% TBWL (3.2% mean difference). Ultimately, 62.1% (lower confidence bound of 59.2%) of treatment participants achieved a 5% TBWL or greater at 24 weeks. At 48 weeks, treated participants who lost weight during the initial 24 weeks using Obalon had maintained 5.7% TBWL on average, whereas control participants were not assessed at the 48-week time point.

AspireAssist gastric emptying device

The AspireAssist enables removal of a portion of stomach contents through a modified gastrostomy tube. The PATHWAY clinical trial for the AspireAssist gastric emptying device was a randomized, nonblinded comparative study.[16] Participants randomized to the treatment group had the AspireAssist device placed and underwent lifestyle therapy consisting of behavior education, diet, and exercise for 12 months. Participants randomized to the control group only underwent lifestyle therapy. At 12 months, treated participants experienced an average 12.1% TBWL, whereas control participants experienced an average 3.6% TBWL (8.5% mean difference). Overall, 58.6% of treated participants achieved 10% or greater TBWL.

Patient-reported outcomes

Patient-reported outcomes (PROs) are also used in assessing device benefits against risks. Determinations regarding how much patients value the treatment, the willingness of patients to take the risk of this treatment to achieve the benefit, the treatment's ability to improve the overall quality of life, and how well patients are able to understand the benefits and risks of the treatments are important factors. **Table 2** lists PROs considered during the clinical studies for the endoscopic weight-loss devices.

All participants in the IB-500 study for the ORBERA IGB reported a significant improvement in the Impact of Weight on Quality of Life-Lite (IWQoL-Lite), which assesses obesity-related quality of life and the Short Form 36 Health Version (SF-36) health survey, which measures general quality of life.[13] However, the ORBERA treatment group had a larger effect size compared with the control group in all domains of the SF-36 at 9 months and in the IWQoL-Lite. Results from the REDUCE trial for the

Table 2
Patient-reported outcome tools evaluated for recently US Food and Drug Administration–approved endoscopic weight-loss devices

PRO Tool	Tool Assessment	Trials Evaluated in
IWQoL-Lite	Obesity-specific QoL	ReShape, ORBERA, and AspireAssist
SF-36	General health-related QoL	ReShape and ORBERA
TFEQ-R18	Cognitive restraint of eating, disinhibition, and hunger	ReShape
Abdominal pain visual analog scale	Abdominal pain	ReShape
Rhodes index of nausea, vomiting, and retching	Nausea, vomiting, and retching	ReShape
Depressive symptoms (BDI-II [Beck Depression Inventory II])	Beck Depression Inventory	ORBERA
Eating behaviors (QEWP-R [Questionnaire on Eating and Weight Patterns-Revised])	Eating attitudes and behaviors	ORBERA and AspireAssist

Abbreviation: QoL, quality of life.

ReShape IGB showed a statistically significant improvement in quality-of-life measures (IWQoL-Lite and SF-36: physical functioning) at 24 weeks for the treated participants as compared with the control participants; these improvements generally persisted in the treated participants to 48 weeks. No differences were seen in other categories of the SF-36 survey or the Three-Factor Eating Questionnaire (TFEQ) between control and treatment participants in the REDUCE trial.[12]

Patient Preference for Endoscopic Weight-Loss Devices

One of CDRH's strategic priorities is to partner with patients to promote a culture of meaningful patient engagement and to increase use and transparency of patient input as evidence in decision making.[45] A Preference Calculator for Weight-Loss Devices (Preference Calculator) tool has been developed to aid in incorporating patient preference into regulatory decision making for devices intended for weight loss.[20] Discrete-choice questions in a scientific survey were used to develop the Preference Calculator tool to provide insight into the amount of risk patients are willing to accept for a given decrease in weight (benefit).

The Preference Calculator tool is intended to answer 3 questions from a patient's perspective:

1. What percentage of patients would prefer getting the device instead of receiving no device?
2. What is the maximum risk that a patient would accept for a given weight loss?
3. What is the minimum benefit that a patient would accept for given risks and impact on eating habits?

The evidence collected via the clinical trials for the endoscopic weight-loss devices was used to develop sample IGB and gastric-emptying device profiles, which are not intended to represent the currently approved obesity devices.

The following considerations were made when developing patient and device profiles used with the Preference Calculator:

- Women made up most of the weight-loss clinical trial participants ($\approx$ 86%–95%). Thus, the authors used weights for 5′4″ women that correlate with BMIs for minimum and maximum indicated device populations.[46]
- Weight loss duration was considered to be the period since device placement through when the weight measurement was taken.
- The mean duration of each reported device- or procedure-related gastrointestinal adverse event was averaged across all reported events to determine the duration of minor side effects.[12–14,16]
- The Preference Calculator allows for discrete choices for chance of side effects requiring hospitalization. Of the choices, the device profile for an IGB and gastric-emptying device includes a 5% no surgery risk associated with device side effects.
- The Preference Calculator offers discrete choices for recommended diet restrictions. An IGB can cause patients to eat a restricted amount at one time and wait a specific time between meals, both of which are device profile options. A gastric-emptying device does not impose any specific dietary restriction on users; however, the AspireAssist has a restricted number of times that it can be used without clinical follow-up. Therefore, the authors conducted the analysis assuming that a $^1/_4$ cup of food eaten at one time and waiting 4 hours between eating are the device profile attributes for IGBs and gastric-emptying devices, respectively (**Table 3**). A sensitivity analysis of the minimum benefit for the dietary restriction

Table 3
Patient preference output from the Preference Calculator reporting the percentage of respondents who would prefer the device over a no-device alternative, what an acceptable minimum benefit would be considering the device profile, and the maximum acceptable mortality risk considering the device profile

		IGB Profile			
		Minimum Indicated BMI (30 kg/m^2)		Maximum Indicated BMI (40 kg/m^2)	
Benefit Duration		6 mo	12 mo	6 mo	12 mo
Respondents judged better than no device, %		6	12	7	13
Minimum benefit (%TBWL)	Average patient	>30	>30	>30	>30
	Risk-tolerant patient	23 (18–29)	21 (17–27)	17 (14–22)	16 (12–20)
Maximum mortality risk (%)	Average patient	0.2 (0.1–0.5)	0.2 (0.1–0.6)	0.2 (0.1–0.5)	0.3 (0.1–0.6)
	Risk-tolerant patient	1.8 (0.8–4.0)	2.3 (1.1–4.8)	2.0 (0.9–4.3)	2.4 (1.2–5.0)

		Gastric-Emptying Device Profile	
		Minimum Indicated BMI (35 kg/m^2)	Maximum Indicated BMI (55 kg/m^2)
Benefit Duration		12 mo	12 mo
Respondents judged better than no device, %		11	22
Minimum benefit (%TBWL)	Average patient	>30	25 (20–32)
	Risk-tolerant patient	20 (16–25)	13 (10–16)
Maximum mortality risk (%)	Average patient	0.3 (0.1–0.6)	0.3 (0.2–0.7)
	Risk-tolerant patient	2.3 (1.1–4.6)	3.4 (1.7–6.5)

95% confidence intervals in parentheses.
%TBWL is not considered relative to a sham or control arm but is absolute.
Upper limit of weight-loss levels included in the study design for the Preference Calculator is 30%.
IGB Profile: 6-month benefit: 8%; 12-month benefit: 6%; dietary restriction: eat $^1/_4$ cup of food at a time; minor side-effect duration: 1 mo; chance of hospitalization: 5%, no surgery; comorbidity: 50% dose/risk.
Gastric-emptying device profile: 12-month benefit: 12%; dietary restriction: wait 4 hours between eating; minor side-effect duration: 2.5 mo; chance of hospitalization: 5%, no surgery; comorbidity: 50% dose/risk.

demonstrates that patients prefer to eat less than to wait in between eating. On average, the minimum acceptable benefit increases by ≈ 1% to 2% when patients have to wait in between meals. Similarly, the maximum acceptable risk decreases by ≈ 0.1% to 0.7%.

- The Preference Calculator has discrete choices for comorbidities. A 50% average reduction in dose of prescription drugs for comorbidity at the lower weight or chance of getting comorbidity most closely aligns with reports from the IGB and gastric-emptying device clinical trials.
- The authors considered a 0% mortality risk associated with the chance of dying from the device within 1 year from receiving the device only. A sensitivity analysis that includes a 0.1% mortality risk associated with having an endoscopic procedure increases the minimum acceptable benefit by 1% for all risk-tolerant patients except those with the highest indicated BMI whose weight loss endures for 12 months.

Using these profiles, IGBs and gastric-emptying devices were evaluated in the Preference Calculator (see **Table 3**). The Preference Calculator provides estimates in the middle 50% and the upper 25% of the sample, which indicate the preferences of average patients and risk-tolerant patients, respectively. The Preference Calculator indicates that average patients with a current or previous BMI of 30 to 40 kg/m^2 who are willing to lose weight would prefer to have a device that can provide at least 30% TBWL for the hypothetical IGB risk profile. In general, 6% to 7% of these patients would prefer an IGB over no device considering the risks and 6-month benefit. Potentially, 12% to 13% of these patients would prefer an IGB over no device considering the 12-month benefit from reviewed clinical trial data; however, the clinical trial data obtained thus far have not evaluated all study participants for a 12-month benefit. Also, 11% to 22% of the patient population would prefer a gastric-emptying device over no device considering the risks and 12-month benefit (see **Table 3**).

Summary

The regulatory perspectives on obesity treatment devices based on the FDA's experience reviewing these devices were discussed. This article also revisited the benefit-risk paradigm FDA offered for consideration when designing a clinical trial for a weight-loss device. The clinical outcomes from the devices discussed here can provide insight to where these devices fit into the current paradigm. As new devices are evaluated, the FDA may work to update the paradigm. In addition, the authors reported on patient weight-loss expectations for 2 generic endoscopic device types using the Preference Calculator.

Moving forward, FDA encourages obesity treatment device manufacturers to seek FDA advice using the Pre-Submission program, which was developed as a means for FDA to provide feedback regarding nonclinical or clinical testing methods used to support premarket submissions.[22] The FDA also believes it is beneficial to submit a Pre-Submission to facilitate early FDA feedback and determine the appropriateness of certain regulatory pathways, such as de novo or PMA. Obesity is an important public health concern, and the consequences of obesity have implications for the health and well-being of the US population.[42,43] FDA recognizes the important impact on public health that new treatments for obesity may have and is committed to the advancement of safe and effective endoscopic devices for the treatment of obesity.

ACKNOWLEDGMENTS

The authors acknowledge Martin Ho, PhD and Telba Irony, PhD for their helpful discussions on the use of the Patient Preference Calculator for Weight-Loss Devices. They also acknowledge Joyce Whang, PhD, Carolyn Neuland, PhD, and Jason Schroeder, PhD for their critical reading of the article and Cynthia Long, MD for comments. In addition, the authors thank Dr Herbert Lerner, MD for his efforts related to obesity treatment device trials and premarket submissions during his tenure with the FDA.

REFERENCES

1. Guh DP, Zhang W, Bansback N, et al. The incidence of co-morbidities related to obesity and overweight: a systematic review and meta-analysis. BMC Public Health 2009;9:88.
2. National Heart Lung and Blood Institute (NHLBI). Managing Overweight and Obesity in Adults, Systematic Evidence Review From the Obesity Expert Panel. 2013. Available at: http://www.nhlbi.nih.gov/sites/www.nhlbi.nih.gov/files/obesity-evidence-review.pdf. Accessed January 3, 2017.

3. Food and Drug Administration. Orlistat (marketed as Alli and Xenical) Information. 2015. Available at: http://www.fda.gov/Drugs/DrugSafety/PostmarketDrugSafety InformationforPatientsandProviders/ucm180076.htm. Accessed January 3, 2017.

4. Food and Drug Administration. FDA approves Belviq to treat overweight or obese adults. 2012. Available at: http://www.fda.gov/NewsEvents/Newsroom/Press Announcements/ucm309993.htm. Accessed January 3, 2017.

5. Food and Drug Administration. FDA approves weight-management drug Qsymia. 2012. Available at: http://www.fda.gov/NewsEvents/Newsroom/Press Announcements/ucm312468.htm. Accessed January 3, 2017.

6. Food and Drug Administration. Naltrexone for extended-release injectable suspension (marketed as Vivitrol) information. 2015. Available at: http://www.fda. gov/Drugs/DrugSafety/PostmarketDrugSafetyInformationforPatientsandProviders/ ucm103334.htm. Accessed January 3, 2017.

7. Food and Drug Administration. FDA approves weight-management drug Saxenda. 2014. Available at: http://www.fda.gov/NewsEvents/Newsroom/Press Announcements/ucm427913.htm. Accessed January 3, 2017.

8. Food and Drug Administration. Summary of Safety and Effectiveness (SSED) REALIZE Adjustable Gastric Band (Model 2200-X). 2007. Available at: http:// www.accessdata.fda.gov/cdrh_docs/pdf7/P070009B.pdf. Accessed January 3, 2017.

9. Food and Drug Administration. Summary of Safety and Effectiveness (SSED) for the LAP-BAND Adjustable Gastric Banding (LAGB) System. 2001. Available at: http://www.accessdata.fda.gov/cdrh_docs/pdf/P000008B.pdf. Accessed January 3, 2017.

10. Goyal D, Watson RR. Endoscopic bariatric therapies. Curr Gastroenterol Rep 2016;18(6):26.

11. Neylan CJ, Dempsey DT, Tewksbury CM, et al. Endoscopic treatments of obesity: a comprehensive review. Surg Obes Relat Dis 2016;12(5):1108–15.

12. Food and Drug Administration. Summary of Safety and Effectiveness Data (SSED) for ReShape Integrated Dual Balloon System. 2015. Available at: http:// www.accessdata.fda.gov/cdrh_docs/pdf14/P140012b.pdf. Accessed January 3, 2017.

13. Food and Drug Administration. Summary of Safety and Effectiveness (SSED) for ORBERA Intragastric Balloon System. 2015. Available at: http://www.accessdata. fda.gov/cdrh_docs/pdf14/P140008b.pdf. Accessed January 3, 2017.

14. Food and Drug Administration. Summary of Safety and Effectiveness (SSED) for Obalon Balloon System. 2016. Available at: http://www.accessdata.fda.gov/ cdrh_docs/pdf16/P160001b.pdf. Accessed January 3, 2017.

15. Food and Drug Administration. Summary of Safety and Effectiveness (SSED) for the MAESTRO Rechargeable System. 2015. Available at: http://www.accessdata. fda.gov/cdrh_docs/pdf13/p130019b.pdf. Accessed January 3, 2017.

16. Food and Drug Administration. Summary of Safety and Effectiveness (SSED) for AspireAssist. 2016. Available at: http://www.accessdata.fda.gov/cdrh_docs/ pdf15/p150024b.pdf. Accessed January 3, 2017.

17. Rohde U, Hedback N, Gluud LL, et al. Effect of the EndoBarrier gastrointestinal liner on obesity and type 2 diabetes: a systematic review and meta-analysis. Diabetes Obes Metab 2016;18(3):300–5.

18. Sandler BJ, Rumbaut R, Swain CP, et al. One-year human experience with a novel endoluminal, endoscopic gastric bypass sleeve for morbid obesity. Surg Endosc 2015;29(11):3298–303.

19. Food and Drug Administration. Patient Preference Information—Voluntary Submission, Review in Premarket Approval Applications, Humanitarian Device Exemption Applications, and De Novo Requests, and Inclusion in Decision Summaries and Device Labeling. 2016. Available at: http://wcms.fda.gov/downloads/MedicalDevices/DeviceRegulationandGuidance/GuidanceDocuments/UCM4466 80.pdf. Accessed January 3, 2017.

20. Ho MP, Gonzalez JM, Lerner HP, et al. Incorporating patient-preference evidence into regulatory decision making. Surg Endosc 2015;29(10):2984–93.

21. Lerner H, Whang J, Nipper R. Benefit-risk paradigm for clinical trial design of obesity devices: FDA proposal. Surg Endosc 2013;27(3):702–7.

22. Food and Drug Administration. Premarket Notification (510k). 2014. Available at: http://www.fda.gov/MedicalDevices/DeviceRegulationandGuidance/Howto MarketYourDevice/PremarketSubmissions/PremarketNotification510k/. Accessed January 3, 2017.

23. Food and Drug Administration. The 510(k) Program: Evaluating Substantial Equivalence in Premarket Notifications [510(k)]. 2014. Available at: http://www.fda.gov/downloads/MedicalDevices/.../UCM284443.pdf. Accessed January 3, 2017.

24. Food and Drug Administration. De Novo Classification Process (Evaluation of Automatic Class III Designation) DRAFT Guidance. 2014. Available at: http://www.fda.gov/downloads/MedicalDevices/DeviceRegulationandGuidance/GuidanceDocuments/UCM273903.pdf. Accessed January 3, 2017.

25. Food and Drug Administration. Factors to Consider When Making Benefit-Risk Determinations in Medical Device Premarket Approval and De Novo Classifications. 2012. Available at: http://www.fda.gov/downloads/MedicalDevices/DeviceRegulationandGuidance/GuidanceDocuments/UCM296379.pdf. Accessed January 3, 2017.

26. Food and Drug Administration. Premarket Approval (PMA). 2014. Available at: http://www.fda.gov/MedicalDevices/DeviceRegulationandGuidance/HowtoMarket YourDevice/PremarketSubmissions/PremarketApprovalPMA/default.htm. Accessed January 3, 2017.

27. Food and Drug Administration. PMA Guidance Documents. 2013. Available at: http://www.fda.gov/MedicalDevices/DeviceRegulationandGuidance/HowtoMarket YourDevice/PremarketSubmissions/PremarketApprovalPMA/ucm143067.htm. Accessed January 3, 2017.

28. Food and Drug Administration. Medical Devices Advisory Committee. Available at: http://www.fda.gov/AdvisoryCommittees/CommitteesMeetingMaterials/Medical Devices/MedicalDevicesAdvisoryCommittee/. Accessed January 3, 2017.

29. Food and Drug Administration. Device Advice: Investigational Device Exemption (IDE). 2014. Available at: http://www.fda.gov/MedicalDevices/DeviceRegulationand Guidance/HowtoMarketYourDevice/InvestigationalDeviceExemptionIDE/. Accessed January 3, 2017.

30. Food and Drug Administration. FDA Decisions for Investigational Device Exemption Clinical Investigations. 2014. Available at: http://www.fda.gov/downloads/medicaldevices/deviceregulationandguidance/guidancedocuments/ucm279107.pdf. Accessed January 3, 2017.

31. Food and Drug Administration. IDE Guidance. 2014. Available at: http://www.fda.gov/MedicalDevices/DeviceRegulationandGuidance/HowtoMarketYourDevice/ucm162453.htm. Accessed January 3, 2017.

32. Gonzalez LM, Moeser AJ, Blikslager AT. Porcine models of digestive disease: the future of large animal translational research. Transl Res 2015;166(1):12–27.

33. Swindle MM, Smith AC. Swine in the laboratory. 3rd edition. Boca Raton (FL): CRC Press; 2016.
34. Ells LJ, Mead E, Atkinson G, et al. Surgery for the treatment of obesity in children and adolescents. Cochrane Database Syst Rev 2015;(6):CD011740.
35. Armstrong S, Lazorick S, Hampl S, et al. Physical examination findings among children and adolescents with obesity: an evidence-based review. Pediatrics 2016;137(2):e20151766.
36. Food and Drug Administration. Premarket Assessment of Pediatric Medical Devices. 2014. Available at: http://www.fda.gov/downloads/MedicalDevices/DeviceRegulationandGuidance/GuidanceDocuments/ucm089742.pdf. Accessed January 3, 2017.
37. Food and Drug Administration. Summary of Pediatric Advisory Committee Meeting. 2005. Available at: http://www.fda.gov/ohrms/dockets/ac/05/minutes/2005-4179m_summary.pdf. Accessed January 3, 2017.
38. Food and Drug Administration. Pediatric Advisory Committee Meeting Documents. Available at: http://www.fda.gov/ohrms/dockets/ac/oc05.html#pediatric. Accessed January 3, 2017.
39. Food and Drug Administration. Pediatric Advisory Committee Meeting, November 17, 2005. 2005. Available at: http://www.fda.gov/ohrms/dockets/ac/05/transcripts/2005-4179t2.pdf. Accessed January 3, 2017.
40. Food and Drug Administration. 2012 Materials of the Gastroenterology-Urology Devices Panel. Available at: http://www.fda.gov/AdvisoryCommittees/CommitteesMeetingMaterials/MedicalDevices/MedicalDevicesAdvisoryCommittee/Gastroenterology-UrologyDevicesPanel/ucm286235.htm. Accessed January 3, 2017.
41. Food and Drug Administration. Guidance for Industry: Developing Products for Weight Management, DRAFT Guidance. 2007. Available at: http://www.fda.gov/downloads/Drugs/.../Guidances/ucm071612.pdf. Accessed January 3, 2017.
42. Jensen MD, Ryan DH, Apovian CM, et al. 2013 AHA/ACC/TOS guideline for the management of overweight and obesity in adults: a report of the American College of Cardiology/American Heart Association Task Force on Practice Guidelines and The Obesity Society. J Am Coll Cardiol 2014;63(25 Pt B):2985–3023.
43. National Institutes of Health. Clinical guidelines on the identification, evaluation, and treatment of overweight and obesity in adults—the evidence report. Obes Res 1998;6(S2):51S–179S.
44. Colman E. Food and Drug Administration's Obesity Drug Guidance Document: a short history. Circulation 2012;125(17):2156–64.
45. Food and Drug Administration. 2016-2017 Strategic Priorities Center for Devices and Radiological Health. 2016. Available at: http://www.fda.gov/downloads/AboutFDA/CentersOffices/OfficeofMedicalProductsandTobacco/CDRH/CDRHVisionandMission/UCM481588.pdf. Accessed January 3, 2017.
46. Ogden CL, Fryar CD, Carroll MD, et al. Mean body weight, height, and body mass index, United States 1960-2002. Adv Data 2004;(347):1–17.
47. EnteroMedics. Instructions for Use. Available at: http://www.accessdata.fda.gov/cdrh_docs/pdf13/P130019C.pdf. Accessed January 3, 2017.

Reimbursement for Endoscopic Bariatric Therapies

Joel V. Brill, MD[a,b,*]

KEYWORDS

- Endoscopy • Bariatric therapies • Reimbursement • Intragastric devices

KEY POINTS

- Intragastric devices may be of benefit to patients who are unable to achieve weight loss through lifestyle modification and pharmaceuticals.
- With the help of every member of a multidisciplinary team and ongoing commitment from patients, small, practical steps and goals can lead to long-lasting, healthy weight loss.

There has been increasing interest in new payment and delivery models designed to improve the effectiveness and efficiency of clinical care. Although efforts have typically focused on improving the management of conditions at a primary care level, there has also been interest in improving care provided by specialists. Over the past several decades, there has been a heightened awareness of the epidemic of obesity. The United States Preventive Service Task Force (USPSTF) recommends screening all adults for obesity. Clinicians should offer or refer patients with a body mass index (BMI) of 30 kg/m^2 or higher to intensive multicomponent behavioral interventions.[1] The USPSTF recommends that clinicians screen children age 6 years and older for obesity and offer or refer them to comprehensive, intensive behavioral interventions to promote improvement in weight status.[2]

Endoscopic or surgical approaches should not be a sole solution to the management of patients with obesity. They are components of a framework that support a multidisciplinary approach to the management of each patient. Providing bariatric endoscopy in the absence of a comprehensive obesity management program benefits no one; not the patient, the patient's family, employer, purchaser, or payer. Thus, it is

Disclosures: Consulting and/or advisory board participation with Endogastric Solutions, FAIR Health, Avella Specialty Pharmacy, Cardinal Health, Eli Lilly, Indivior Pharmaceuticals, Braeburn Pharmaceuticals, OrexoUS, Halt Medical, Bayer, Natera, Nestle Health Sciences, AstraZeneca, Blue Earth Diagnostics, Vermillion, Medtronic. Consulting and options in EndoChoice, Gene-News, SynerZ. Governing board and options in SonarMD.
[a] Predictive Health LLC, Paradise Valley, AZ, USA; [b] University of Arizona College of Medicine, Tucson, AZ, USA
* 3639 E. Denton Lane, Paradise Valley, AZ 85253.
E-mail address: joel.brill@gmail.com

Gastrointest Endoscopy Clin N Am 27 (2017) 343–351
http://dx.doi.org/10.1016/j.giec.2017.01.002
1052-5157/17/© 2017 Elsevier Inc. All rights reserved.

giendo.theclinics.com

crucial for practices that wish to provide bariatric endoscopic services to ensure that the patients have access to other services across multiple disciplines that, taken together, support the management of obesity, which is a chronic disease.

CODING ENDOSCOPIC PLACEMENT AND REMOVAL OF GASTRIC DEVICES FOR THE MANAGEMENT OF OBESITY

Available clinical data and manufacturer recommendations indicate 6 months to be the current standard duration of therapy for the intragastric balloon (IGB) devices approved by the US Food and Drug Administration (FDA) as of January 1, 2017.

The ORBERA Intragastric Balloon System is indicated for use as an adjunct to weight reduction for adults with obesity with a BMI of greater than or equal to 30 and less than or equal to 40 kg/m^2 and is to be used in conjunction with a long-term supervised diet and behavior modification program designed to increase the possibility of significant long-term weight loss and maintenance of that weight loss. ORBERA is indicated for adult patients who have failed more conservative weight reduction alternatives, such as supervised diet, exercise, and behavior modification programs.[3]

The ReShape Integrated Dual Balloon System is indicated for weight reduction when used in conjunction with diet and exercise in patients with a BMI of 30 to 40 kg/m^2 and 1 or more obesity-related comorbid conditions. It is indicated for use in adult patients who have failed weight reduction with diet and exercise alone.[4]

The Obalon Balloon System is a swallowable intragastric balloon system indicated for temporary use to facilitate weight loss in adults with obesity (BMI of 30–40 kg/m^2) who have failed to lose weight through diet and exercise. The system is intended to be used as an adjunct to a moderate-intensity diet and behavior modification program.[5]

At present, there are no CPT (Current Procedural Terminology) or HCPCS (Healthcare Common Procedural Coding System) codes for the endoscopic placement of intragastric space-occupying or gastric pacing devices for the management of obesity. Endoscopic placement should be reported using code 43999 (unlisted procedure, stomach). Nonendoscopic placement of an intragastric space-occupying device should be reported using code 99199 (unlisted special service, procedure, or report). Endoscopic removal of a foreign body from the stomach should be reported using code 43247 (esophagogastroduodenoscopy, flexible, transoral; with removal of foreign body or bodies).

The AspireAssist is intended to assist in weight reduction of patients with obesity. It is indicated for use in adults aged 22 years or older with a BMI of 35.0 to 55.0 kg/m^2 who have failed to achieve and maintain weight loss with nonsurgical weight loss therapy. The AspireAssist is intended for a long-term duration of use in conjunction with lifestyle therapy and continuous medical monitoring.[6]

Endoscopic placement of a percutaneous gastrostomy-type device for the management of obesity should be reported using code 43246 (esophagogastroduodenoscopy, flexible, transoral; with directed placement of percutaneous gastrostomy tube). If the device is placed under fluoroscopic guidance without endoscopic visualization, the service would be reported using code 49440 (insertion of gastrostomy tube, percutaneous, under fluoroscopic guidance including contrast injections, image documentation, and report).

Endoscopic removal of a percutaneous gastrostomy-type device for the management of obesity should be reported using code 43247. If the device is removed as part of an evaluation and management (EM) visit, only the EM code is reported. If the device is removed endoscopically and replaced endoscopically, then code 43247 should be used to report removal, and code 43246 to report endoscopic placement of a subsequent percutaneous gastrostomy-type device. If the device is replaced without imaging or endoscopic guidance, then code 43760 (percutaneous change of gastrostomy tube without imaging or endoscopic guidance) is appropriate. If the device is replaced under fluoroscopic guidance, then code 49450 (replacement of gastrostomy under fluoroscopic guidance) is appropriate.

The manufacturers of the endoscopic devices require the endoscopist to participate in an endoscopic-skills training program before the company will sell the device to the physician. The physician must show advanced upper endoscopy skill and experience by possession of interventional endoscopy privileges granted locally by the participating hospital or ambulatory facility. Physicians are required to use the device as a component of a multidisciplinary weight management practice that provides appropriate endoscopy facilities, nutrition and exercise counseling, psychological and radiological support, and long-term support and follow-up.

There are no requirements specifying that placement and/or removal of endoscopic devices for obesity always require general anesthesia and/or intubation.[7] Orotracheal intubation is recommended in patients with BMI greater than 40 kg/m^2, and in those with obstructive sleep apnea or chronic obstructive pulmonary disease. Some endoscopists elect to perform the initial placement of the device using general anesthesia and airway intubation. Endoscopic removal of IGB devices must be completed in the presence of an empty stomach, and patients should be nil per os (NPO) for a minimum of 12 hours before removal. A strict gastric emptying protocol is recommended 48 hours before the patient is due to undergo the balloon removal procedure. Some experienced endoscopists recommend that the airway be protected from aspiration of acid or gastric contents dripping from the IGB for the first several balloon removals, especially if the endoscopist does not frequently remove large foreign bodies from the stomach. If food is found in the stomach on endoscopic examination, then measures (aspiration of stomach contents, endotracheal intubation, or delay of procedure) must be taken to protect the airway.[8] Risks, potential complications, and side effects of intragastric devices should be discussed with the patient before proceeding with placement.[9]

COMPLICATIONS RELATED TO GASTRIC DEVICES FOR THE MANAGEMENT OF OBESITY

Risks, potential complications, and side effects of intragastric devices should be discussed with the patient before proceeding with placement.[9] The manufacturers of the space-occupying devices have noted 2 absolute contraindications to the use of these devices:

- The presence of more than 1 intragastric device at the same time.
- Prior open or laparoscopic stomach or bariatric surgery.

In addition, there are several relative contraindications to be considered when considering placement of an IGB:

- Any inflammatory disease of the gastrointestinal tract, including esophagitis, gastric ulceration, duodenal ulceration, cancer, or specific inflammation, such as Crohn disease.
- Potential upper gastrointestinal bleeding conditions, such as esophageal or gastric varices, congenital or acquired intestinal telangiectasia, or other congenital anomalies of the gastrointestinal tract, such as atresias or stenoses.
- A large hiatal hernia or greater than 5-cm hernia or less than or equal to 5 cm with associated severe or intractable gastroesophageal reflux symptoms.
- A structural abnormality in the esophagus or pharynx, such as a stricture or diverticulum that could impede passage of the delivery catheter and/or an endoscope.
- Achalasia or any other severe motility disorder that may pose a safety risk during removal of the device.

- Gastric mass.
- Severe coagulopathy.
- Hepatic insufficiency or cirrhosis.
- Patients who are known or suspected to have an allergic reaction to materials contained in the intragastric device.
- Any other medical condition that would not permit elective endoscopy, such as poor general health or history and/or symptoms of severe renal, hepatic, cardiac, and/or pulmonary disease.
- Uncontrolled mental disorder or a neurodevelopmental disorder that could compromise patient understanding of, or compliance with, follow-up visits and removal of the device after 6 months.
- Recent or current eating disorder, including but not limited to self-induced vomiting.
- Recent or current substance use disorder.
- Patients who are unable or unwilling to take prescribed proton pump inhibitor medication for the duration of the device implant.
- Patients unwilling to participate in an established medically supervised diet and behavior modification program, with routine medical follow-up.
- Patients receiving aspirin, antiinflammatory agents, anticoagulants, or other gastric irritants, not under medical supervision.
- Patients who are known to be pregnant or breast feeding.
- Patients who lack a general understanding about the procedure, risks, benefits, expected outcomes, and the necessary lifestyle changes recommended.

For patients considering IGB devices that contain methylene blue, patients receiving serotonergic drugs, including selective serotonin reuptake inhibitors, serotonin norepinephrine reuptake inhibitors, monoamine oxidase inhibitors, and other prescription and over-the-counter drugs, should be cautioned about the possibility of developing serotonin syndrome because of the combination of these medications and the release of methylene blue (in the event of balloon rupture). Patients should immediately seek medical attention if they develop any symptoms of confusion, headache, nausea and vomiting, rapid heart rate, or severe sweating.

The risk of obstructions may be higher in patients who have diabetes, a dysmotility disorder, or who have had prior abdominal or gynecologic surgery. Patients with known abdominal adhesions or who have had prior abdominal surgery or any signs or symptoms of a bowel obstruction should be carefully evaluated before use of these devices in relation to possible intestinal obstruction should the device deflate or pass into the intestines. Bowel obstructions have been reported to be caused by deflated balloons passing into the intestines and have required surgical removal. The patient's clinical history should be considered when assessing the suitability of the patient and the risk of the procedure.

To prevent ulcers, it is recommended that the patient start a program of oral proton pump inhibitors (PPIs) for approximately 3 to 5 days before placement so that a maximal gastric acid suppression effect will be present on the day of placement. It is recommended that the PPI dose be given sublingually if nausea and/or vomiting are present. An oral PPI with the highest recommended starting dose (eg, omeprazole 40 mg daily or equivalent) should be continued as long as the device is in place.

It is recommended that no food or liquid is present in the stomach at the time of the insertion procedure. Representative preprocedure diet instructions include:

- Forty-eight hours before the procedure: soft food only, no meat in any form
- Twenty-four hours before the procedure: clear liquids only
- Twelve hours before the procedure: no food or liquids by mouth

For removal, clear liquids for a minimum of 24 hours, and preferably 48 hours, is recommended, because there is significant documented delay in gastric emptying with the IGB device in place.[10,11] Several experienced gastroenterologists also recommend ingestion of a clear, carbonated, low-calorie beverage between 12 and 24 hours before the procedure to clean the surface of the balloon before removal.

Endoscopic removal of IGB devices must be completed in the presence of an empty stomach. Patients should be NPO for a minimum of 12 hours before removal. If food is found in the stomach on endoscopic examination, then measures (aspiration of stomach contents, endotracheal intubation, or delay of procedure) must be taken to protect the airway. In the event of an emergency removal by a physician untrained in the procedure, endotracheal intubation of the patient is recommended to reduce the risk of aspiration, because the risk of aspiration of gastric contents into the patient's lungs is serious and may lead to death.

Patients reporting loss of satiety, increased hunger, and/or weight gain should be evaluated expeditiously because this may indicate a balloon deflation. Physical examination, plain abdominal radiograph, upper gastrointestinal examination, and endoscopy can be helpful in confirming the diagnosis. Deflated devices should be removed promptly. Patients should be advised that balloon deflation may lead to serious adverse events, including bowel obstruction and need for emergency surgery.

Possible complications of IGB placement include:
- Intestinal obstruction by the balloon.
- Death caused by complications related to intestinal obstruction.
- Esophageal obstruction.
- Gastric outlet obstruction.
- Injury to the digestive tract during placement of the balloon in an improper location, such as in the esophagus or duodenum.
- Insufficient or no weight loss.
- Adverse health consequences resulting from weight loss.
- Gastric discomfort and feelings of nausea and vomiting following balloon placement as the digestive system adjusts to the presence of the balloon.
- Continuing nausea and vomiting.
- Abdominal or back pain, either steady or cyclic.
- Gastroesophageal reflux.
- Influence on digestion of food.
- Blockage of food entering into the stomach.

The percutaneous gastric aspiration device has a unique set of contraindications and complications. Contraindications include:
- Previous abdominal surgery that significantly increases the medical risks of gastrostomy tube placement.
- Esophageal stricture, pseudo-obstruction, severe gastroparesis, or gastric outlet obstruction.
- Inflammatory bowel disease.
- History of refractory gastric ulcers.
- Ulcers, bleeding lesions, or tumors discovered during endoscopic examination.
- Uncontrolled hypertension (blood pressure >160/100 mm Hg).
- History or evidence of serious pulmonary or cardiovascular disease, including acute coronary syndrome, heart failure requiring medications, or New York Heart Association (NYHA) class III or IV.

- Coagulation disorders (platelet count <50,000/μL, prothrombin time >2 seconds more than control, or International Normalized Ratio >1.5).
- Anemia (hemoglobin level <8.0 g/dL in women and <10.0 g/dL in men).
- Pregnant or lactating.
- Diagnosed bulimia or diagnosed binge-eating disorder (using Diagnostic and Statistical Manual of Mental Disorders criteria).
- Night eating syndrome.
- Chronic abdominal pain that would potentially complicate the management of the device.
- Physical or mental disability, or psychological illness that could interfere with compliance with the therapy.
- At high risk of having a medical complication from the endoscopic procedure or a weight loss program for any reason, including poor general health or severe organ dysfunction such as cirrhosis or renal dysfunction.

Possible adverse events of the gastrostomy tube device include:

- Peristomal granulation tissue
- Abdominal pain and discomfort after device placement
- Nausea, vomiting
- Dyspepsia, acid reflux, heartburn, hiccups, belching
- Peristomal irritation, inflammation, discharge
- Peristomal bacterial or fungal infection
- Peristomal bleeding
- Hypokalemia
- Change in bowel habits, constipation, diarrhea
- Accidental dislodgement or trauma to the device

DATA COLLECTION

Practitioners who provide endoscopic placement of devices for the management of obesity should collect data on the efficacy of interventions. The devices currently available have been approved by the FDA with fewer than 300 patients in each of the pivotal studies. With a target population of more than 60 million patients with obesity, it is the responsibility of the end user to assist in further defining the results and potential adverse events that can be discovered when applying an invasive therapy to a large population. At a minimum, data collection should include[12,13]:

- Demographic elements
  - Age, gender, race, ethnicity
- Vital signs
  - Blood pressure, height, weight
- Anthropometric elements
  - BMI, waist/hip ratio, bioelectrical impedance, skinfold measures
- Medical history/Review of Status (ROS)
  - Presence/duration of comorbid conditions
  - Medication use; for weight loss, other diseases/conditions
  - Use of supplements, alcohol, tobacco, illicit substances
- Endoscopic history
  - Patient's medical status and weight history before and at device placement
  - Physician, dietitian, behaviorist visits (before and during device placement)
  - Device placement; complications; admissions/readmissions; death
  - Device duration/date of device removal

- ○ Emergency room visits
- ○ Adjuvant medications used during/after device placement
- Weight history
  - ○ Birth weight
  - ○ Age at onset of overweight/obesity
  - ○ Duration of overweight/obesity
  - ○ When and by whom was overweight/obesity first recognized
  - ○ Dietitian visits
  - ○ Number, speed, and duration of prior weight loss attempts; outcomes
  - ○ Helpers/barriers to success (causative factors, contributors)
- Typical food intake/behaviors
  - ○ Macronutrients (ie, protein, fat, carbohydrates)
  - ○ Micronutrients (vitamins/minerals)
  - ○ Timing/frequency of meals/snacks
- Psychosocial elements
  - ○ Presence of/association with adverse childhood experiences
  - ○ Home environment: 2 parents plus siblings; divorce, death, single family, step-parent/siblings, grandparents, adoption, and so forth
  - ○ Behaviorist visits (prior/current)
  - ○ Behavior modification attempts (prior/current)
  - ○ Readiness to change
- Economic elements
  - ○ Homeless, food assistance, and so forth
- Physical activity
  - ○ Type, amount, frequency (prior/current/after device placement)
- Strategies to facilitate weight loss (desired outcomes)
  - ○ Food/activity records routinely kept
  - ○ Improved diet quality/patterns of food consumption
  - ○ Reduced carbohydrate, calorie, fat consumption
  - ○ Increased physical activity
  - ○ Follow-up appointments routinely kept
  - ○ Health status/weight assessed and recorded at 1 month, 6 months, and 12-month intervals after device placement (minimum)
  - ○ Weight loss and maintenance of loss at 12 months and yearly postprocedure
  - ○ Improvement in 1 or more obesity-associated comorbidities; eg, hypertension, diabetes, hyperlipidemia
  - ○ Dosage reduction and/or elimination of 1 or more medications associated with treatment of obesity-associated comorbidities

INTERNATIONAL STATISTICAL CLASSIFICATION OF DISEASES AND RELATED HEALTH PROBLEMS, 10TH REVISION, CODES FOR OBESITY

As of October 1, 2015, International Statistical Classification of Diseases and Related Health Problems, 10th Revision (ICD-10), codes should be used when submitting claims for professional services. The pertinent ICD-10 codes for obesity are:

- E66: overweight and obesity
- Use additional code to identify BMI, if known (eg, Z68.3)

E66: overweight and obesity
  E66.0: obesity caused by excess calories
    E66.01: morbid (severe) obesity caused by excess calories

E66.09: Other obesity caused by excess calories
E66.1: drug-induced obesity
E66.2: morbid (severe) obesity with alveolar hypoventilation
E66.3: overweight
E66.8: other obesity
E66.9: obesity, unspecified

BMI adult codes are for use for persons 21 years of age or older. BMI pediatric codes are for use for persons 2 to 20 years of age. These percentiles are based on the growth charts published by the Centers for Disease Control and Prevention.

Z68: BMI
Z68.3: BMI 30 to 39, adult
Z68.30: BMI 30.0 to 30.9, adult
Z68.31: BMI 31.0 to 31.9, adult
Z68.32: BMI 32.0 to 32.9, adult
Z68.33: BMI 33.0 to 33.9, adult
Z68.34: BMI 34.0 to 34.9, adult
Z68.35: BMI 35.0 to 35.9, adult
Z68.36: BMI 36.0 to 36.9, adult
Z68.37: BMI 37.0 to 37.9, adult
Z68.38: BMI 38.0 to 38.9, adult
Z68.39: BMI 39.0 to 39.9, adult
Z68.4: BMI 40 or greater, adult
Z68.41: BMI 40.0 to 44.9, adult
Z68.42: BMI 45.0 to 49.9, adult
Z68.43: BMI 50.0 to 59.9, adult
Z68.44: BMI 60.0 to 69.9, adult
Z68.5: BMI pediatric
Z68.51: less than fifth percentile for age
Z68.52: fifth percentile to less than 85th percentile for age
Z68.53: 85th percentile to less than 95th percentile for age
Z68.54: greater than or equal to 95th percentile for age

SUMMARY

Intragastric devices may be of benefit to patients who are unable to achieve weight loss through lifestyle modification and pharmaceuticals. With the help of every member of a multidisciplinary team and ongoing commitment from patients, small, practical steps and goals can lead to long-lasting, healthy weight loss.[14]

REFERENCES

1. LeBlanc E, O'Connor E, Whitlock EP, et al. Screening for and management of obesity and overweight in adults. Evidence report no. 89. AHRQ publication no. 11-05159-EF-1. Rockville (MD): Agency for Healthcare Research and Quality; 2011.
2. Whitlock EP, O'Connor EA, Williams SB, et al. Effectiveness of primary care interventions for weight management in children and adolescents: an updated, targeted systematic review for the USPSTF. Evidence synthesis no. 76. AHRQ publication no. 10-05144-EF-1. Rockville (MD): Agency for Healthcare Research and Quality; 2010.

3. Orbera Intragastric Balloon System. Directions for use. Available at: http://www. orbera.com/resource/1464712622000/o_orbera_code/pdf/ORBERA_Directions_ for_Use_GRF-00346-00R01.pdf. Accessed December 28, 2016.
4. ReShape Medical. Instructions for use. Available at: https://reshapeready. com/wp-content/uploads/2015/07/ReShape_Instructions_For_Use.pdf. Accessed December 28, 2016.
5. Obalon Balloon System. Directions for use. Available at: http://www.obalon.com/ wp-content/uploads/2016/12/P160001.Obalon.BalloonIFU.PhysicianLabeling.IR-10_Response_clean_0908201612.pdf. Accessed December 28, 2016.
6. Aspire Assist. Clinician guide. Available at: http://www.aspirebariatrics.com/wp-content/uploads/AspireAssist-Clinician-Guide.pdf. Accessed December 28, 2016.
7. Messina T, Genco A, Favaro R, et al. Intragastric balloon positioning and removal: sedation or general anesthesia? Surg Endosc 2011;25(12):3811–4.
8. Genco A, López-Nava G, Wahlen C, et al. Multi-centre European experience with intragastric balloon in overweight populations: 13 years of experience. Obes Surg 2013;23(4):515–21.
9. Evans JT, DeLegge MH. Intragastric balloon therapy in the management of obesity: why the bad wrap? JPEN J Parenter Enteral Nutr 2011;35(1):25–31.
10. Bonazzi P, Petrelli MD, Lorenzini I, et al. Gastric emptying and intragastric balloon in obese patients. Eur Rev Med Pharmacol Sci 2005;9(5 Suppl 1):15–21.
11. Mion F, Napoléon B, Roman S, et al. Effects of intragastric balloon on gastric emptying and plasma ghrelin levels in non-morbid obese patients. Obes Surg 2005;15(4):510–6.
12. Thomas JG, Bond DS, Phelan S, et al. Weight-loss maintenance for 10 years in the National Weight Control Registry. Am J Prev Med 2014;46(1):17–23.
13. Dayyeh BKA, Kumar N, Edmundowicz SA, et al. ASGE Bariatric Endoscopy Task Force systematic review and meta-analysis assessing the ASGE PIVI thresholds for adopting endoscopic bariatric therapies. Gastrointest Endosc 2015;82(3): 425–38.e5.
14. Blackburn GL, Greenberg I, McNamara A, et al. The multi-disciplinary approach to weight loss: defining the roles of the necessary providers. Bariatric Times June 9 2008. Available at: http://bariatrictimes.com/the-multidisciplinary-approach-to-weight-loss-defining-the-roles-of-the-necessary-providers/. Accessed December 28, 2016.

Moving?

Make sure your subscription moves with you!

To notify us of your new address, find your **Clinics Account Number** (located on your mailing label above your name), and contact customer service at:

Email: journalscustomerservice-usa@elsevier.com

800-654-2452 (subscribers in the U.S. & Canada)
314-447-8871 (subscribers outside of the U.S. & Canada)

Fax number: 314-447-8029

Elsevier Health Sciences Division
Subscription Customer Service
3251 Riverport Lane
Maryland Heights, MO 63043

Printed and bound by CPI Group (UK) Ltd, Croydon, CR0 4YY

08/05/2025

01864699-0008